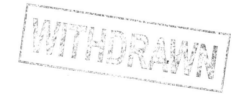

Molecular Diagnosis of Cancer

METHODS IN MOLECULAR MEDICINE™

John M. Walker, SERIES EDITOR

Molecular Diagnosis of Cancer, edited by *Finbarr E. Cotter,* 1996

Human Cell Culture Protocols, edited by *Gareth E. Jones,* 1996

Antisense Therapeutics, edited by *Sudhir Agrawal,* 1996

Vaccine Protocols, edited by *Andrew Robinson, Graham H. Farrar, and Christopher N. Wiblin,* 1996

Prion Diseases, edited by *Harry F. Baker and Rosalind M. Ridley,* 1996

Molecular Diagnosis of Genetic Diseases, edited by *Rob Elles,* 1996

Herpes Simplex Virus Protocols, edited by *Moira S. Brown and Alasdair MacLean,* 1996

Helicobacter pylori **Protocols,** edited by *Christopher L. Clayton and Harry T. Mobley,* 1996

Lectins in Medical Research, edited by *Jonathan M. Rhodes and Jeremy D. Milton,* 1996

Gene Therapy Protocols, edited by *Paul Robbins,* 1996

METHODS IN MOLECULAR MEDICINE™

Molecular Diagnosis of Cancer

Edited by

Finbarr E. Cotter

University of London, UK

Humana Press ✳ **Totowa, New Jersey**

© 1996 Humana Press Inc.
999 Riverview Drive, Suite 208
Totowa, New Jersey 07512

This publication is printed on acid-free paper. ∞
ANSI Z39.48-1984 (American Standards Institute) Permanence of Paper for Printed Library Materials.

Cover illustration: Fig. 1 from Chapter 6, "Polymerase Chain Reaction for Detection of the t(14;18) Translocation in Lymphomas," by Peter W. M. Johnson.

Photocopy Authorization Policy:

Printed in the United States of America. 10 9 8 7 6 5 4 3 2 1

Library of Congress Cataloging in Publication Data

Main entry under title:

Methods in molecular medicine™.

Molecular diagnosis of cancer / edited by Finbarr E. Cotter.
      p. cm. — (Methods in molecular medicine)
   Includes index.
   ISBN 0-89603-341-4 (alk. paper)
   1. Cancer—Molecular diagnosis. I. Cotter, Finbarr E.
II. Series.
   [DNLM: 1. Neoplasms—diagnosis. 2. DNA—analysis. 3. Polymerase
Chain Reaction. 4. Genetic Techniques. QZ 241 M7173 1996]
RC270.M64 1996
616.99'4075—dc20
DNLM/DLC
for Library of Congress   96-20789
                                          CIP

Preface

The aims of *Molecular Diagnosis of Cancer* are to introduce scientists and physicians working in the field of diagnostics to the area of cancer molecular pathology and to highlight the possibilities of its application to the cancer physician in the clinic. The degree of molecular biological expertise required should be minimal, although those with more experience may also be able to benefit from the book. All of the authors have considerable practical experience in the method they describe and are working predominantly in the setting of the cancer clinic. As such, the book pulls together a number of techniques that are already being applied to a wide range of malignancies. Moreover, this field will continue to expand exponentially as further research leads to a greater understanding of the molecular basis of cancer.

Detection of the changes to the DNA or RNA code within a diseased cell often provides pathological information for the diagnosis, prognosis, and management of the disease. Such DNA-related analysis is primarily the role of molecular pathology. Methods to detect these alterations are being refined and are evolving from the research to the diagnostic laboratory. One of the single most powerful techniques in this new branch of pathology has been the polymerase chain reaction (PCR), to which much of this book is devoted. The use of PCR in pathology not only provides new diagnostic possibilities, but also requires the acquisition of new expertise in its performance and in interpretation of the results if the full potential is to be achieved.

PCR is an in vitro technique, invented by Kary Mullis, that produces multiple copies of selected sequences of DNA, provided the sequence is present in the test DNA sample. Its sensitivity lies in the region of a million-fold amplification from a template equivalent of as little as a single human cell and, for this reason, rigorous methods to minimize and control for contamination are required. An important property of PCR when considering diagnostic applications is the ability of the method to amplify from target DNA sequences not only those well prepared from freshly frozen tissue, but also those from degraded DNA templates, such as those found in paraffin-embedded tissue.

Amplification by PCR is ideally suited to target sequences of DNA below 1000 bases in size, above which the efficiency of the reaction falls dramatically. However, lengthening the extension time for the reaction can yield longer amplification products. Specificity of the reaction is influenced by several factors. Excess of *Taq* polymerase, excessive extension times, and low annealing temperatures will all increase the risk of spurious amplification; however, the opposite approach leads to greater specificity, with the penalty of a reduced quantity of amplification product. PCR initially leads to an exponential accumulation of DNA, but a plateau of amplification product is eventually reached (ideally after 25 cycles). Further amplification within the plateau phase may lead to accumulation of detectable product from low levels of contaminant DNA. Essentially, less rather than more cycles may, ironically, be optimal in PCR.

Often, the gene sequences that are required to be detected consist of a number of exon sequences separated by long intron regions. DNA PCR would not be possible because the distance between the primers is too great. However, nature normally splices out the intron sequence when producing mRNA, bringing the exon sequences considerably closer. If the mRNA is extracted and converted back into complementary DNA (reverse transcription [RT] to cDNA), then this would permit PCR, as described above, to use the exon primers, as they are much closer. This process (RT-PCR) is useful for the examination of quite large pieces of DNA, such as chromosomal translocation, in which the DNA breakpoints are varied and over a large distance but the resultant chimeric fusion gene remains constant. The use of PCR in molecular diagnostics of cancer primarily uses the RT methodology and has been applied predominantly in the field of hematological malignances, in which chromosomal translocations leading to the presence of chimeric genes are observed in many cases. The abundance of molecular diagnostic methods in blood malignancies in part reflects the relative ease of examination, which results from the accessibility of the "tumor" cell from the bone marrow and its presence in a cell suspension.

Identification of cancers associated with mutations in gene sequences requires detection of as little as a single base sequence difference. Single-strand conformation polymorphism (SSCP) analysis is a quick and effective technique, based on PCR, for the detection of single nucleotide base substitutions. The method relies on the principle that single-stranded DNA takes on sequenced-based secondary structures (Conformers) under nondenaturing conditions. In real terms, this means that molecules varying by as little as a single base substitution may form different conformers and migrate differently in a nondenaturing polyacrylamide gel. The best results are obtained when the DNA molecule being examined is 200 base pairs or less in size. SSCP analysis for a base mutation is carried by PCR using flanking oligonucleotide primers (commonly to a gene sequence) and incorporating a [^{35}S] or [^{32}P] labeled dATP in the reaction. The radioactive PCR product is made single stranded by boiling and is then run on the denaturing gel. The polyacrylamide gel is then dried and exposed to an autoradiograph to show the presence or absence of a base mutation. Directly sequencing the PCR product by the dideoxy method (to confirm correct amplification and the presence of mutations suggested by SSCP) can be executed in the thermal cycler by a method known as cycle sequencing, directly incorporating radioactivity. The application of SSCP is predominantly in the area of solid tumors and is usually suggestive of a tumor suppressor gene, illustrated well by the P53 and Wilm's tumor genes.

There are two major problems related to PCR, namely the false positive and the false negative results. These drawbacks can be largely overcome provided adequate care and good positive and negative control reactions are carried out at all times with this extremely sensitive technique.

False Positive. Those arising by this contamination constitute a very serious problem. Minute numbers of cells containing equivalent amounts of DNA, often transferred by contaminated syringes, pipet tubes, tubes, or gloves, may be readily amplified and cause problems with the interpretation of results. Only the most stringent precautions taken while collecting and manipulating samples, together with positive and negative controls (reaction mixes with no DNA, or DNA known to be negative or positive for the set of primers used), will help avoid false positive results. Precautions include physically isolating PCR preparations and PCR product, autoclaving of solutions, UV irradiating solutions, aliquoting reagents, using disposable gloves, avoiding splashes and using positive displacement pipets, premixing reagents, and adding the test DNA last.

False Negative. Positive and negative controls remain as important when determining the possibility of a false negative result. The true false negative means that the target DNA was present in the test DNA, but was not detected in the PCR reaction. This may be caused by sampling errors in which the target sequence for PCR was present in very low numbers in the tissue DNA extracted. The quantity of DNA taken for the reaction would not always be adequate to contain a PCR target sequence. Poor quality of DNA may also be a problem. These can be guarded against by using PCR with known primers that readily amplify human DNA to judge the quality of the DNA for PCR, whereas multiple testing will help exclude low levels of disease as a cause for the negative result. RT-PCR raises another problem concerning the false negative result, which may be owing to a "resting" cell that is temporarily not expressing the disease-related gene. Here, the failure to detect the positive result does not exclude its subsequent detection and should be considered when interpreting RT-PCR results. The last element to be considered is the negative result with such consensus primers as those used in antigen receptor PCR, in which clonal evolution by the disease may lead to a negative result, or the consensus is inadequate to give good annealing for PCR. Essentially, if results raise doubts, then repeat the PCR.

As a technique, PCR has now had eight years of development. Modifications of the basic method in the field of cancer have now provided a sensitive and flexible approach to the provision number of diagnostic possibilities, including sequences analysis, detection of base mutations, demonstration of chimeric gene products, and the determination of the presence or absence of altered DNA related to disease. In the next few years, there will be a further expansion with enzymatic amplification becoming even more automated and entering the routine pathology laboratories to improve our understanding and management of cancer.

Recently, a number of less sensitive but just as powerful techniques, including fluorescence *in situ* hybridization (FISH), a modification called comparative genome hybridization (CGH), the detection of apoptosis (programmed cell death), and *in situ* hybridization (ISH), have added to the molecular diagnostic repertoire. The methodology for these newer methods is given in the final chapters of this book.

It is our hope that workers in the field of cancer molecular pathology will be able to use the practical guides given to initiate and evaluate cancer patients and will also be able to use the experience gained to further develop their molecular diagnostic skills as further consistent DNA alterations are discovered in tumor material.

Finbarr E. Cotter

Contents

Preface v

Contributors xi

List of Color Plates xiii

PART I. HEMATOLOGICAL MALIGNANCIES

1 PCR of Gene Rearrangements for the Detection of Minimal Residual
   Disease in Childhood ALL,
   **Nick Goulden, Kenneth Langlands, Colin Steward, Chris Knechtli,
   Mike Potter, and Tony Oakhill** 3

2 Detection of BCR-ABL in Hematological Malignancies by RT-PCR,
   Nicholas C. P. Cross 25

3 Molecular Diagnosis of Acute Myeloid Leukemia with Maturation,
   FAB-Type M2,
   Ewald J. B. M. Mensink and Louis T. F. van de Locht 37

4 Analysis of the PML/RAR-α Fusion Gene in Acute Promyelocytic
   Leukemia by Reverse-Transcription Polymerase Chain Reaction:
   Technical Recommendations, Advantages, and Pitfalls,
   **Daniela Diverio, Anna Luciano, Roberta Riccioni,
   Francesco Lo Coco, and Andrea Biondi** 47

5 RT-PCR Analysis of Breakpoints Involving the MLL Gene Located
   at 11q23 in Acute Leukemia,
   Chris F. E. Pocock and Finbarr E. Cotter 55

6 Polymerase Chain Reaction for Detection of the t(14;18) Translocation
   in Lymphomas,
   Peter W. M. Johnson 63

7 NPM-ALK Reverse Transcriptase-Polymerase Chain Reaction Analysis
   for Detection of the t(2;5) Translocation of Non-Hodgkin's Lymphoma,
   Sheila A. Shurtleff, James R. Downing, and Stephan W. Morris 75

8 Molecular Diagnosis of the 5q Deletion in Malignant Myeloid Disorders,
   Jackie Boultwood 91

9 Polymerase Chain Reaction Based Methods for Assessing Chimerism
   Following Allogeneic Bone Marrow Transplantation,
   Mark Lawler and Shaun R. McCann 105

PART II. SOLID TUMORS

10 Identification of Mutations in the Retinoblastoma Gene,
    Annette Hogg *123*

11 Mutational Analysis of the Wilms' Tumor (WTI) Gene,
    Linda King-Underwood and Kathy Pritchard-Jones *141*

PART III. GENERAL TECHNIQUES FOR CANCER ANALYSIS

12 Single-Strand Conformation Polymorphism Mutation Analysis
    of the p53 Gene,
    Mark J. Booth *151*

13 The Characterization of Chromosomal Abnormalities Using
    Fluorescence *In Situ* Hybridization Procedures,
    Helena M. Kempski *161*

14 Comparative Genomic Hybridization,
    Briana J. Williams *183*

15 *In Situ* Hybridization of Cells and Tissue Sections,
    Simon J. Conway *193*

16 Apoptosis Detection by DNA Analysis,
    Paul D. Allen and Adrian C. Newland *207*

Index *215*

Contributors

PAUL D. ALLEN • *Department of Haematology, London Medical College, London, UK*

ANDREA BIONDI • *Clinica Pediatrica, Università di Milano, Ospedale S. Gerardo, Monza, Italy*

MARK J. BOOTH • *LRF Department of Haematology and Oncology, Institute of Child Health, University of London, UK*

JACKIE BOULTWOOD • *LRF Molecular and Cytogenetic Haematology Unit, Department of Haematology, John Radcliffe Hospital, Oxford, UK*

SIMON J. CONWAY • *Division of Cell and Molecular Biology, The Institute of Child Health, University of London, UK*

FINBARR E. COTTER • *LRF Department of Haematology and Oncology, Institute of Child Health, University of London, UK*

NICHOLAS C. P. CROSS • *LRF Centre for Adult Leukaemia, Royal Postgraduate Medical School, London, UK*

DANIELA DIVERIO • *Dipartimento di Biopatologia, Divisione di Ematologia, Università "La Sapienza," Roma, Italy*

JAMES R. DOWNING • *Department of Tumor Cell Biology, St. Jude Children's Research Hospital, Memphis, TN*

NICK GOULDEN • *Department of Pathology and Microbiology, University of Bristol, UK*

ANNETTE HOGG • *The Hanson Centre for Cancer Research, Adelaide, Australia*

PETER W. M. JOHNSON • *ICRF Cancer Medicine Research Unit, St. James University Hospital, Leeds, UK*

HELENA M. KEMPSKI • *LRF Centre for Childhood Leukaemia, Department of Molecular Haematology, Institute of Child Health, London, UK*

LINDA KING-UNDERWOOD • *Section of Paediatrics, Institute of Cancer Research, Sutton, UK*

CHRIS KNECHTLI • *Department of Pathology and Microbiology, University of Bristol, UK*

KENNETH LANGLANDS • *Department of Pathology and Microbiology, University of Bristol, UK*

MARK LAWLER • *Sir Patrick Dun Research Laboratory, Department of Haematology and Oncology, St. James Hospital and Trinity College, Dublin, Ireland*

FRANCESCO LO COCO • *Dipartimento di Biopatologia, Divisione di Ematologia, Università "La Sapienza," Roma, Italy*

ANNA LUCIANO • *Clinica Pediatrica, Università di Milano, Ospedale S. Gerardo, Monza, Italy*

SHAUN R. MCCANN • *Sir Patrick Dun Research Laboratory, Department of Haematology and Oncology, St. James Hospital and Trinity College, Dublin, Ireland*

EWALD J. B. M. MENSINK • *Division of Haematology and Central Haematology Laboratory, University Hospital Nijmegen, Nijmegen, The Netherlands*

STEPHAN W. MORRIS • *Department of Experimental Oncology, St. Jude Children's Research Hospital, Memphis, TN*

ADRIAN C. NEWLAND • *Department of Haematology, London Medical College, London, UK*

TONY OAKHILL • *Department of Pathology and Microbiology, University of Bristol, UK*

CHRIS F. E. POCOCK • *LRF Department of Haematology and Oncology, Institute of Child Health, University of London, UK*

MIKE POTTER • *Department of Pathology and Microbiology, University of Bristol, UK*

KATHY PRITCHARD-JONES • *Section of Paediatrics, Institute of Cancer Research, Sutton, UK*

ROBERTA RICCIONI • *Clinica Pediatrica, Università di Milano, Ospedale S. Gerardo, Monza, Italy*

SHEILA A. SHURTLEFF • *Department of Pathology, St. Jude Children's Research Hospital, Memphis, TN*

COLIN STEWARD • *Department of Pathology and Microbiology, University of Bristol, UK*

LOUIS T. F. VAN DE LOCHT • *Division of Haematology and Central Haematology Laboratory, University Hospital Nijmegen, Nijmegen, The Netherlands*

BRIANA J. WILLIAMS • *Departments of Pediatrics and Human Genetics, Eccles Institute of Human Genetics, University of Utah, Salt Lake City, UT*

List of Color Plates

Color plates appear as an insert following p. 178.

Plate 1 (Fig. 4 from Chapter 13). The application of whole chromosome paints for the identification of chromosome rearrangement.

Plate 2 (Fig. 8 from Chapter 13). Interphase cells from a patient with chronic myelogenous leukemia.

Plate 3 (Fig. 11 from Chapter 13). Centromeric probes used following a sex-mismatched bone marrow transplant.

Plate 4 (Fig. 5 from Chapter 13). Alpha-satellite centromeric probes used for detection of aneuploidy in interphase cells.

Plate 5 (Fig. 6 from Chapter 13). Phage, cosmid, and YAC probes.

Plate 6 (Fig. 9 from Chapter 13). The detection of loss of heterozygosity in retinoblastoma.

Plate 7 (Fig. 10 from Chapter 13). The detection of loss of heterozygosity in Wilms' tumor.

Plate 8 (Fig. 1 from Chapter 14). Comparative genomic hybridization of a prostate cancer xenograft, LuCAP; and an inverse DAPI (pseudo-Geisma binding) image of the same metaphase for chromosome identification.

I

HEMATOLOGICAL MALIGNANCIES

1

PCR of Gene Rearrangements for the Detection of Minimal Residual Disease in Childhood ALL

Nick Goulden, Kenneth Langlands, Colin Steward, Chris Knechtli, Mike Potter, and Tony Oakhill

1. Introduction

The study of submicroscopic or minimal residual disease (MRD) in childhood acute lymphoblastic leukemia may eventually lead to stratification of therapy on an individual patient basis (reviewed in ref. *1*). PCR of immunoglobulin heavy chain (IgH) and T-cell receptor (TCR) gene rearrangements provides widely informative markers (Table 1), which, in the majority of cases, are stable during the disease course *(2)*. Generation of leukemia-specific probes using this technique allows detection of MRD at levels of one leukemic cell in 10,000 to 100,000 normal bone marrow mononuclear cells (BM MNC).

The genes that encode antibody and T-cell receptors provide immense diversity. They are arranged into three families called variable (V), diversity (D), and joining (J) regions. The process of gene rearrangement during normal lymphocyte development recombines random V, D, and J segments resulting in a clone-specific DNA sequence. A more detailed description of this can be found in Steward et al., 1993 *(3)*.

Leukemic cells can be thought of as the clonal progeny of a single lymphocyte that has undergone neoplastic transformation during normal development. In the majority of acute lymphoblastic leukemia (ALL), the leukemic cells have rearranged their receptor genes prior to diagnosis. As leukemic cells completely replace the normal BM architecture at presentation, clone-specific gene rearrangements can be identified by PCR from marrow DNA obtained at this time. These can subsequently be used as probes for detection of residual disease *(4–6)*. It should be noted that lineage infidelity occurs in acute leukemia,

From: *Methods in Molecular Medicine, Molecular Diagnosis of Cancer*
Edited by: F. E. Cotter Humana Press Inc., Totowa, NJ

3

Table 1
Primer Systems[a]

Locus	No[b]	Primer sense (ref.)	No[b]	Primer antisense (ref.)	[Mg²⁺]	Size, bp	+B	+T–
IgH FR3	1	5'-ACACGGC(C/T)(G/C)TGTATTACTGT-3' (2)	3	5'-GTGACCAGGGT(C/T)C C(C/T)TGGCCCCAG-3' (2)	1.5–3.0	65-155	75%	8%
			4	5'-AACTGCAGAGGAGACGGTGACC-3' (3)	1.5–3.0	80-170		
			2	5'-GACCAGGGT(C/T)C C(C/T)TGGCCCCAG-3' [c]				
Vδ2-Dδ3	5	5'-CTTGCACCATCAGAGAGAGA-3' (2)	7	5'-GTTTTTGTACAGGTCTCTGT-3'	1.0–3.0	100-150	45%	4%
			8	5'-AGGGAAATGGCACTTTTGCC-3' (2)	1.5–3.0	110-170		
			6	5'-TTTTGTACAGGTCTCTGT-3' [c]				
Vδ1-Jδ1		5'-GCCTTACAGCTAGAAGATTC-3'		5'-GTTCCTTTTCCAAAGATGAG-3'	1.5–3.0	80-150	5%	25%
Vγ1-Jγ1/2[d]		5'-TG(A/C)(C/T)TCTGG(A/G)GTCTATTACTGT-3'		5'-CGATACTTACCTGTGACAAC(C/A)AG-3'	3.0	80-160	45%[d]	90%[d]
VγII-Jγ1/2[d]		5'-AAACAGGACATAGCTACCTACT-3'		5'-CGATACTTACCTGTGACAACC/AAG-3'	3.0	80-160	45%[d]	90%[d]
lead Vδ2-anti Vδ2		5'-GTCATGTCAGCCATTGAGTT-3'		5'-TCTCTCTCTGATGGTGCAAG-3'	1.5	220	control	control

[a] The primers shown here use a common buffer and generate products that can easily be resolved on 8% PAGE. [b] Refers to Fig. 1. [c] Sequencing primers. The Vγ1 primer is a consensus primer and amplifies all members of this group except Vγ7. + B and +T [d] These primers can be used in a multiplex reaction. indicate the percentage of patients by lineage expected to show a clonal rearrangement at each locus at diagnosis.

2.5.3. Generation of Single-Stranded Template

1. 0.1*M* NaOH (5*M* stock, freshly prepared).
2. 2X B&W buffer (*see* Section 2.5.1.).
3. 1X PCR buffer (*see* Section 2.1.).

2.5.4. Cycle Sequencing

2.5.4.1. END LABELING OF SEQUENCING PRIMER

1. Primer: 1 m*M* stock.
2. 10X T4 end labeling buffer (manufacturer's specification).
3. T4 polynucleotide kinase (10 U/reaction).
4. γ^{33}P dATP (10 mCi–1 μL/reaction).
5. Distilled water.

2.5.4.2. PREPARATION OF SEQUENCING BULK MIX

1. 10X *Taq* polymerase buffer (PCR buffer).
2. 25 m*M* dNTP mix.
3. *Taq* polymerase (0.5 U/μL).
4. Distilled water.
5. 20 μL from completed end labeling reaction (*see* Section 2.6., item 1).

2.5.4.3. PREPARATION OF TERMINATION REACTIONS

500-μL Eppendorf tubes as follows:

1. Template DNA.
2. Sequencing bulk mix (*see* Section 2.6., item 2).
3. Dideoxy nucleotide triphosphate (ddNTP) stock solution: ddATP 1 m*M*, ddCTP 1 m*M*, ddGTP 500 μ*M* or ddTTP 2 m*M*.
4. Mineral oil.
5. Formamide loading dye: 90% formamide, 0.25% bromophenol blue, 0.25% xylene cyanol, and 1 m*M* EDTA.
6. 6% denaturing PAGE gel.
7. 10% methanol/10% acetic acid mixture.
8. Hyperfilm β-max X-ray film (Amersham) RT.

2.6. PCR for Detection of Residual Disease

1. "Outer primer" (*see* Table 1).
2. Bulk "master reaction mix" as in Section 2.2.1.
3. Normal control bone marrow (BM) mononuclear cell (MNC) DNA.
4. 8% PAGE gel.

2.7. Detection of Low-Level Residual Disease by Allele-Specific Hybridization

Two methods exist for this (*see* Note 7).

2.7.1. Dot Blotting

1. Dot blot manifold.
2. Vacuum pump.
3. 5 μL of PCR product diluted to 100 μL in 2X SSC (*see* Section 2.7.2., item 7).
4. Hybond N$^+$ nylon membrane (Amersham).
5. 2X SSC: 0.3M sodium chloride, 0.1M sodium citrate.
6. Whatman 3M blotting paper.
7. 0.4M NaOH.
8. Laboratory clear film.

2.7.2. Electroblot Analysis

1. Electroblot apparatus (e.g., Millipore electroblot apparatus).
2. 1-mm thick 8% PAGE gel.
3. 1X TBE (*see* Section 2.3.).
4. Ethidium bromide (10 mg/mL).
5. Whatman 3M filter paper.
6. Hybond N$^+$ nylon membrane (Amersham).
7. 2X SSC: 0.3M sodium chloride, 0.1M sodium citrate.
8. 0.4M NaOH.
9. Laboratory clear film.

2.7.3. Hybridization of Allele-Specific Probes to Membranes

2.7.3.1. LABELING OF PROBES

1. Oligonucleotide probes (1 mM conc.).
2. γ^{32}P dATP using the protocol described in Section 3.5.4.1. (*see* Note 16).
3. End-labeling solutions (*see* Section 2.5.4.1.).
4. Patient Product Probes.
5. Hexamer labeling solutions (*see* Section 2.4.2.).

2.7.3.2. HYBRIDIZATION

1. Hybridization buffer (e.g., Rapid Hybridization buffer, Amersham).
2. Labeled probe.

2.7.4. Washing

1. 6X SSC (made from 20X stock consisting of 3M sodium chloride, 1M sodium citrate).
2. 2X SSC.
3. 0.1X SSC/1% SDS.
4. Laboratory clear film
5. X-ray film (Hyperfilm MP, Amersham). Store at 4°C.

3. Methods

The method we describe consists of four main steps.

1. Presentation DNA is screened for a clonal rearrangement by PCR as described in Section 3.1., 3.2., and 3.3. Using a combination of IgH, Vδ2-Dδ3 and VγI-II-Jγ1/2 PCR, we are able to amplify at least one rearrangement in 90% of B-lineage ALL. A combination of Vδ1-Jδ1 and VγI/II-Jγ1/2 PCR likewise amplifies at least one rearrangement in 90% of T-ALL (Table 1).

2. A clone-specific probe is generated as described in Sections 3.4. and 3.5. A number of methods are described for the generation of clone-specific probes. In the simplest, clonal PCR products are purified and directly radiolabeled for use as probes (Sections 3.4.1. and 3.4.2.). However, the inclusion of common primer sequences can significantly compromise probe sensitivity. This can be overcome in some cases by removal of the common primer sequence by restriction endonuclease digestion (Section 3.4.3.). The "gold standard" approach is the generation of sequence-specific oligonucleotide probes (Section 3.5.). Although this is technically more complex, in our experience, this is the only method to provide consistent detection of low-level residual disease in all patients.

3. Remission marrow DNA is PCR amplified and transferred to a nylon membrane as described in Sections 3.6. and 3.7. Detection of low-level MRD is based on junction-specific hybridization of leukemic probes to PCR products from marrow taken at the time of apparent remission. Generally 1 µg of remission BM MNC DNA, representing 150,000 cells, is amplified at the appropriate locus. All products are then transferred to a nylon membrane prior to hybridization. Two techniques can be used for transfer; we will discuss these in turn.

4. This membrane is probed with the patient-specific probe as described in Section 3.7. An example of a series of patient samples that have been probed is shown, and guidelines for accurate interpretation of results are provided.

3.1. Screening of Presentation DNA

A total of 0.1 to 1 µg of presentation MNC DNA should be screened by the appropriate locus (*see* Note 2). Presentation DNA can also be obtained from archival slides as described below in Section 3.1.1. (*see* Note 8).

3.1.1. Preparation of Slide DNA for PCR

1. Scrape off a small area (1 cm²) of slide under PBS using a glass Pasteur pipet and transfer to an Eppendorf tube.
2. Spin at full speed in a microfuge for 1 min and discard supernatant.
3. Resuspend pellet in 20 µL 1X PCR buffer and overlay with mineral oil.
4. Heat to 94°C for 10 min.
5. Spin full speed 1 min.
6. Use 2 µL of the supernatant for each PCR taking care not to transfer any cellular material.
7. Prior to reuse, these samples should be heated to 94°C again.

3.2. PCR Protocol

Pay strict attention to possible sources of contamination (*see* Note 9) and keep all reagents on ice. As far as possible, minimize the length of time that the polymerase is out of the freezer. Ensure that all the reagents and template DNA are to hand before starting to set up the reaction. It is advisable to keep primers in small aliquots (<50 mL) to minimize freeze-thawing, which leads to degradation.

3.2.1. Preparation of 100 µL PCR Reactions

1. Take appropriate number of clearly marked 500-µL Eppendorf tubes.
2. Add 50 µL light mineral oil to each tube.
3. Add 96 µL from the bulk "master mix" (Section 2.2.1.) to each tube.
4. Add template DNA (4 µL).
5. Prepare at least one nontemplate DNA containing control.
6. Flick tubes to mix, pulse spin, and transfer to PCR cycler.

3.2.2. PCR Cycler Parameters

All the described primer systems are optimized at the following conditions:

1. Initial denaturation: 94°C for 3 min;
2. 35 cycles of 94°C for 1 min, 55°C for 1 min, and 72°C for 1 min; and
3. Final extension step of 72°C for 5 min.

3.3. Analysis of PCR Products by 8% PAGE (see Note 4)

1. An 8% acrylamide is made. For 80 mL of gel solution, the following ingredients are mixed: 56 mL water, 8 mL 10X TBE, and 16 mL 40% acrylamide stock. 40 µL of TEMED and 300 µL of 10% ammonium persulfate is added immediately before pouring the gel. Once it is fully polymerized, the gel is put at 4°C overnight, along with the required amount of 1X TBE for the gel electrophoresis tank.
2. To each sample, add 1/5 vol of 6X loading buffer.
3. Load 30–40 µL of sample onto the gel.
4. Resolve at 10 V/cm for 3 h at ambient temperature.
5. Stain with ethidium bromide for 5 min.
6. Rinse in 1X TBE prior to visualization on a UV light box.
7. Photograph (A typical PAGE gel showing amplification products from patients with clonal rearrangements and normal polyclonal BM MNC DNA is shown in Fig. 1).

3.4. Direct Generation of Clone-Specific Probes from PCR Products

3.4.1. Elution of DNA from 8% PAGE Gels

1. After ethidium bromide staining, carefully excise bands with a clean razor blade, taking care not to transfer excess acrylamide.
2. Place gel slice in a 500-µL Eppendorf tube with a pierced bottom.

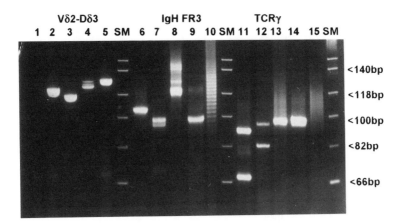

Fig. 1. PAGE analysis of multi-locus gene rearrangements PCR. SM size marker. *Hin*fI digested φX174 DNA is run as a molecular weight size marker. This is essential in discriminating amplification products in the correct size range, allowing identification of primer-dimer or higher molecular weight artifacts. Lanes 1–5, Vδ2-Dδ3 PCR; lane 1, product from 1 mg normal control DNA, which generates a faint polyclonal smear; lanes 2–5, leukemic presentation DNA from four patients showing clear clonal bands. In lane 4, multiple bands are seen reflecting heteroduplex formation as a consequence of biallelic rearrangement. Lanes 6–10, IgH FR3-JPS PCR; lane 10, product from 1 μg normal control DNA which generates a polyclonal 3-bp stepladder reflecting normal in-frame rearrangments. Lanes 6–9, amplification of presentation DNAs. Multiple bands may be seen as a consequence of biallelic and secondary gene rearrangement events *(3)*. Lanes 11–15, TCRγ PCR; lane 15, polyclonal smear from product from 1 μg normal control DNA. Lanes 11–14, amplification of presentation DNAs showing clonal bands.

3. Place this tube inside a 1.5-mL Eppendorf tube and spin at full speed in a microfuge for 10 s to generate a finely crushed acrylamide slurry.
4. Suspend slurry in 200 μL of TE (pH 8.0) and incubate overnight at 37°C.
5. Spin at full speed for 5 min and transfer 100 μL of supernatant to a fresh tube, taking care not to transfer particles of acrylamide.
6. Add 50 μL 7.5*M* ammonium sulfate, followed by 300 μL 100% ethanol.
7. Transfer to −70°C 1 h or −20°C overnight.
8. Spin at full speed for 5 min, and discard the supernatant.
9. Wash pellet of DNA and salt in 100 μL of 70% ethanol.
10. Spin at full speed for 10 s and discard supernatant, to leave the DNA pellet.
11. Dry the pellet (air drying is usually adequate) and then resuspend 20 μL TE (pH 7.6).

3.4.2. Labeling (see Note 5)

1. Each labeling reaction should be prepared by mixing the following: 5 μL DNA (approx 25 ng) prepared in Section 3.4.1. and 9 μL distilled water.

2. Boil for 3 min, incubate 2 min on ice and then pulse spin in a microfuge.
3. Add the following, on ice: 2 μL hexamer, 1 μL Klenow, 2 μL buffer/dNTP mix (Random Prime Labeling Kit, Amersham), and 1 μL α^{32}P dCTP.
4. Mix and incubate at 37°C for 30 min.
5. Unincorporated nucleotides are not removed.
6. Denature probes by boiling and keep on ice prior to hybridization.

3.4.3. Preparation of Digested IgH Probes (see Note 6)

1. Take 20 μL presentation PCR product without loading dye (or 10 μL of eluted product DNA, *see* Section 3.4.1.).
2. Mix with the following: 4 μL 10X *Sau* 96 I buffer, 2 μL *Sau* 96 I enzyme, and distilled water to a total volume of 40 μL.
3. Incubate 37°C for 60 min.
4. Resolve both cut and uncut bands by 8% PAGE. The digested probe will be approx 20 bp shorter than the uncut version.
5. Excise, precipitate, and label the cut band as in Sections 3.4.1. and 3.4.2.

3.5. Generation of Sequence-Specific Oligonucleotide Probes

This requires template preparation for solid-phase sequencing of presentation rearrangements (*see* Note 10). Presentation products generated with a biotinylated primer are required (*see* Note 11). Phases are separated by a Dynal magnetic particle separator (MPS-E) at each stage.

3.5.1. Preparation of Templates
from Monoclonal Rearrangements

1. Wash 20 μL streptavidin M 280 Dynabeads once in 2X B&W buffer.
2. Resuspend in 40 μL B&W buffer.
3. Mix with 40 μL PCR amplification product. This ensures a Na^+ concentration of 1M.
4. Incubate at room temperature (RT) for 15 min with occasional mixing.
5. Remove supernatant using the magnet.
6. Wash beads once in 40 μL 2X B&W.
7. Remove supernatant using the magnet.
8. Proceed as described under generation of single stranded template (*see* Section 3.5.3.).

3.5.2. Preparation from Multiple Rearrangements

1. Elute individual bands from acrylamide gels into 200 μL TE (pH 8.0) as described (*see* Section 3.4.1.).
2. Wash 20 μL streptavidin coated Dynabeads once in 2X B&W buffer.
3. Resuspend beads in 100 μL of 2X B&W buffer and mix with an equal volume of eluate.
4. Incubate RT for 15 min.
5. Remove supernatant using the magnet.
6. Wash beads once in 40 μL of 2X B&W.

7. Remove supernatant using the magnet.
8. Proceed as described under generation of single stranded template (*see* Section 3.5.3.).

3.5.3. Generation of Single-Stranded Template

1. Add 8 µL 0.1*M* NaOH.
2. Incubate at room temperature for 10 min.
3. Remove the supernatant (keeping it as this contains the complementary strand).
4. Wash the beads in 40 µL of 0.1*M* NaOH, followed by 40 µL of 2X B&W buffer.
5. Resuspend in 45 µL of 1X PCR buffer.

3.5.4. Cycle Sequencing

This protocol was modified from Murray, 1989 (7).

3.5.4.1. END LABELING OF SEQUENCING PRIMER (*see* NOTE 11)

1. Mix the following: 2 µL primer, 2 µL 10X end-labeling buffer, 1 µL T4 polynucleotide kinase, 1 µL γ^{33}P dATP, and 14 µL distilled water.
2. Incubate at 37°C for 30 min.

3.5.4.2. PREPARATION OF SEQUENCING BULK MIX

Mix: 20 µL end-labeling reaction, 56 µL 10X *Taq* polymerase buffer, 56 µL dNTP mix, 14 µL *Taq* polymerase, and 24 µL distilled water. This provides sufficient mix to sequence seven different bands.

3.5.4.3. PREPARATION OF TERMINATION REACTIONS

1. Four termination reactions (A, C, G, or T) are prepared for each band being sequenced. These are prepared in 500-µL Eppendorf tubes as follows: 10 µL template DNA, 6 µL sequencing bulk mix, and 4 µL of the appropriate dideoxy nucleotide triphosphate (ddNTP) stock solution
2. Overlay each reaction with mineral oil and perform 15 PCR cycles of 94°C, 55°C, 72°C for 1 min each.
3. Add 6 µL formamide loading dye.
4. Denature at 80°C for 3 min, then snap-cool on ice.
5. Resolve 5-µL aliquots on 6% denaturing PAGE gels run at approx 55°C.
6. Fix for a minimum of 10 min in 10% methanol/10% acetic acid.
7. After drying, autoradiography is performed for 1–3 d with Hyperfilm β-max film (Amersham) at RT without intensification (*see* Note 12).

3.5.5. Probe Design

The specificity of each rearrangement for the detection of leukemia is conferred by junctional sequence. Oligonucleotide probes should therefore span this junctional area. To ensure against nonspecific genomic hybridization-oligoprobes should be at least 17 bases in length. At loci with a single junctional region, TCR Vδ2-Dδ3 and TCRγ, design of oligonucleotide probes spanning this junction is straightforward. TCR Vδ1-Jδ1 rearrangements possess multiple N regions and a choice of the best probe can be made by avoiding long runs of G or C nucleotides and a low melting temperature (resulting from a GC content of less than 40%).

At the IgH locus, there are two junctional regions, but additional considerations influence optimal probe selection. Although multiple bands can be seen at presentation, these arise most often as a consequence of secondary gene rearrangement and share the same DNJ sequence. True oligoclonality that is the presence of more than two unique DNJ segments is rare in our experience. We therefore design probes to each unique DNJ sequence observed at presentation rather than each band. The possibility of false negative disease assessment owing to instability of the IgH locus during the course of disease can also be obviated by this approach in all but 10% of cases *(2)*.

3.6. PCR for the Detection
of Residual Disease in Remission Samples

One microgram of DNA (representing 150,000 cells) prepared from BM MNC collected at presentation and subsequent time points throughout the course of disease are amplified. One microgram of normal BM MNC DNA, a reaction containing no template DNA, and logarithmic dilutions of leukemic DNA in normal DNA are coamplified in order to monitor background, assess contamination, and to provide semiquantitation, respectively (*see* Note 13).

3.6.1. Preparation of Logarithmic Dilutions

1. Concentration of presentation leukemic DNA is assessed by optical density (OD) at 260 nm.
2. DNA is diluted to 0.005 mg/mL. 2 μL of this mix provides the 10^{-2} dilution point (approx 1500 genomes).
3. Serial tenfold dilutions in distilled water are prepared. Mixing is promoted by incubating DNA solutions at 37°C for 30 min between admixes.
4. Dilutions continue until the 10^{-5} (1 copy) or 10^{-6} (0.1 copies) point is reached.

3.6.2. PCR of Remission Samples and Dilutions

1. This should be performed using "outer" primer systems at the appropriate locus if possible (*see* Note 14).
2. Set up the bulk reaction mix as in Section 2.1.1.
3. PCR 1 μg of each remission sample and the two normal controls.
4. For the dilutions, combine 1 μg of normal control BM MNC DNA with 2 μL of each of the logarithmic dilution points.
5. PCR 2 μL of neat (i.e., noncompeted)10^{-4} and 10^{-5} dilutions to check copy number.
6. **Important:** Aim to set up all these reactions at the same sitting to maximize uniformity and minimize contamination.
7. Resolve a 30-μL aliquot of the products on 8% PAGE to check that the reactions have worked. This will also provide a gross assessment of disease load.

3.7. Detection of Low-Level Residual Disease by Allele-Specific Hybridization

Prior to hybridization against leukemia-specific probes, products must be transferred to nylon membrane and denatured. Two methods exist for this and are discussed in Note 7.

3.7.1. Dot Blotting

This is the simplest method, providing rapid screening. It is a useful first line assay. We use a dot blot manifold.

1. Dilute 5 µL PCR product to 100 µL in 2X SSC. It is not necessary to remove the oil from PCR reactions.
2. Presoak an appropriately sized nylon membrane (Hybond N+, Amersham) 5 min 2X SSC (*see* Note 15).
3. Assemble dot blot manifold in the following order:
   a. Base: Whatman 3M blotting paper pad cut to size of membrane and presoaked immediately prior to application. Nylon membrane: top.
   b. Tighten bolts carefully: hand tight only.
   c. Dot samples and apply vacuum until wells drained.
   d. Disassemble blotter before removing vacuum.
   e. Fix and denature DNA by soaking in $0.4M$ NaOH for 1 min.
   f. Neutralize in 2X SSC for 15 s.
   g. Air dry membrane.
   h. Store wrapped in laboratory film at 4°C prior to hybridization.

3.7.2. Electroblot Analysis (see Note 15)

1. Resolve products on 1 mm thick 8% PAGE gels run at 10 V/cm for 3 h in 1X TBE.
2. Stain in ethidium bromide and view under UV.
3. Rinse gel in 1X TBE.
4. Trim gels to 14 × 8 cm and leave to soak in 1X TBE.
5. DNA is now electrophoretically transferred to Hybond-N+ membranes with a semidry Millipore electroblot apparatus. Pads are prepared from Whatman 3M filter paper and presoaked in 1X TBE immediately prior to use.
6. Trim membrane to 12 × 7 cm. Presoak in 1X TBE for 5 min.
7. Overlay bottom (positive) electrode with two Whatman pads, cut to 16 × 10 cm.
8. Overlay pads with nylon membrane.
9. Place gel on top of membrane.
10. Repeated repositioning of the gel should be avoided in order to minimize capillary transfer.
11. Overlay the gel with two additional Whatman pads cut to 12 × 7 cm. This "pyramid" assembly promotes consistent transfer.
12. Assemble blotter and apply a constant current of 4 mA cm-2 (approx 350 mA) for 30 min.
13. Fix, neutralize, and dry membranes as for dot blotting (*see* Section 3.7.1.).
14. Restain gels with ethidium bromide to check transfer (*see* Note 16).

3.7.3. Hybridization of Allele-Specific Probes to Membranes

3.7.3.1. LABELING OF PROBES

1. Oligonucleotide probes: End label 2 μL of a 1 μ*M* oligonucleotide solution with γ^{32}P dATP using the protocol described in Section 3.5.4.1. (*see* Note 17).
2. Patient Product Probes: Label as described in Section 3.4.2.

3.7.3.2. HYBRIDIZATION

1. Prehybridize membranes for 60 min in 5 mL hybridization buffer (e.g., Rapid Hybridization buffer, Amersham) at the calculated hybridization temperature (*see* Note 18).
2. Add probe (>10^6 dpm/μL prehybridization solution) and incubate for an additional hour in the same solution at the same temperature.

3.7.4. Washing

1. Discard probe and rinse membranes in 6X SSC. Probe can be retained for further use at this point.
2. Agitate at room temperature in fresh 6X SSC, two times for 10 min. This usually provides sufficient washing for oligoprobes, and membranes can be sealed in laboratory film ready for autoradiography.
3. If subsequent washes are required (e.g., if probing dot blots). If product probes are used or if high backgrounds are obtained, a further 20 min wash in 2X SSC at the hybridization temperature can be performed.
4. Stringency can be increased to 0.1X SSC/1% SDS at the hybridization temperature and membranes washed until background signals minimized (*see* Note 19).
5. Autoradiography is performed at –70°C with intensification for 4 to 16 h against X-ray film.
6. If necessary, further washes can be performed after autoradiography to improve specificity. It is imperative that membranes are kept moist, if further washes are to be performed.

3.8. Reprobing Membranes

If membranes are to be reprobed, e.g., with an oligonucleotide derived from a second allele, then old probes can be removed by plunging the membrane into 0.5% SDS at 100°C. Allow the solution to cool and remove the membrane after 20 min. Again, it is imperative that membranes are not allowed to desiccate. Nylon membranes can be reprobed several times without diminution of sensitivity.

3.9. Interpretation of Autoradiographs

MRD is detected at low level by sequence-specific hybridization. At maximal sensitivity, clone-specific probes can discriminate the presence of leukemic junctional sequence in a background of other nonleukemic sequences at a level equivalent to the presence of one leukemic cell in 100,000 normals. The specificity of probe binding is influenced by the hybridization temperature, salt concentration in the buffer, probe length, and probe constitution. Of particular concern in the detection of MRD by gene rearrangement PCR, is the presence of shared sequence between the leukemia-specific probe and normal rearrangements. As a result of the above factors, short oligonucleotide probes designed to hybridize to the leukemia-specific junctional region and lacking common primer sequence are optimal. A single base mismatch with this kind of probe results in a drop in melting temperature by 5°C *(11)*.

However, as DNA will always bind nonspecifically to other DNA species, and some common sequence is shared between normal background polyclonal rearrangements and any probe, some degree of nonspecific hybridization to normals always occurs. Interpretation of autoradiographs therefore is dependent on discrimination between the degree of hybridization of the specific probe to remission DNA compared to that seen in the normal controls. In addition, semiquantitative assessment of both the level of probe sensitivity and any residual disease detected can be obtained by examining the dilutions. At low levels of disease, particularly if insensitive probes are used, discrimination by eye alone may be difficult. The use of densitometry could theoretically be employed. This is an equally subjective method. We do not use this technique.

We have illustrated the method and potential pitfalls of interpreting autoradiographs in Fig. 2. This shows a dot blot (A) and an electroblot (B) generated from a series of IgH amplification products. These are derived from BM MNC DNA obtained at various times of remission from a patient suffering from B-lineage ALL.

Figure 2B shows a dot blot of products hybridized with a $\gamma^{32}P$ end-labeled DNJ region oligonucleotide probe. The normal controls N1-N3 are found on the bottom row of the dot blot. By comparing the relative strength of hybridization of the probe between the normals and other specimens the following can be seen. There is copy in both the neat 10^{-4} and 10^{-5} dilutions and the probe is sensitive to 10^{-4} in normal; no hybridization is seen in the non-DNA lane (C). MRD at the 10^{-4} level or greater is seen in samples 1,7, and 8. There is as suggestion of MRD in samples 2, 3, and possibly 4.

Duplicate samples electroblotted then probed with the DNJ probe as above are shown in Fig. 2A. If we consider the dilutions first, we can see that the additional size discrimination provided by electrophoresis prior to probing allows more confident detection of low-level disease. This approach reveals the probe to be sensitive at the 10^{-5} level. In the patient samples, MRD is seen in sample 1, 3, 4, 7, and 8, and also at low level in sample 2.

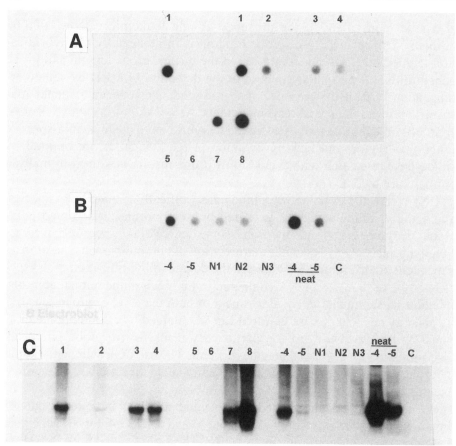

Fig. 2. Comparison of dot and electroblot analysis. **(A)** 8% nondenaturing PAGE gel showing amplified BM DNA samples collected at presentation; d 28, BM harvest (BMH), and at 3, 6, 12, and 18 mo post-BMT. Logarithmic dilutions of tumor DNA in normal BM DNA (10^{-2} to 10^{-5}), normal BM DNA (N), and a no template DNA control (C) are included. **(B)** Dot blot analysis of duplicate products hybridized with α^{32}P labeled 20-base oligonucleotide DNJ region probe. **(C)** Electroblot analysis. Products were resolved by 8% nondenaturing PAGE and electrophoretically transferred to nylon membranes. The second band observed in the dilution lanes is artifactual and does not compromise residual disease assessment.

Dot blots provide a useful first screening method but do not give confident detection of low-level MRD. At times of polyclonal lymphocytosis seen in remission samples after the end of treatment or BMT, nonspecific hybridization of the probe to the products generated by this expanded normal population can lead to false positive MRD detection *(10)*. Therefore, we routinely use the electroblot approach.

Table 2
Troubleshooting

Problem	Probable cause	Solution
Poor probe incorporation	Old isotope	Use fresh isotope (<2 wk old)
	Degraded oligo	Use fresh aliquot of oligo
Blank or faint autoradiographs	Poor probe incorporation	*see* above
	Poor transfer (if electroblot)	Check blotter setup
	Hybridization temperature too high	Check melting temperature
	Incorrect probe sequence	Check sequence
High background	Hybridization temperature too low	Check melting temperature
	Insufficient washing	Increase stringency
	Little probe diversity	Accept reduced sensitivity
		Use alternative locus
Low sensitivity	Poor dilutions	Check copy number
	see Blank or faint autoradiographs	
	High backgrounds	*see* above
Bands in all lanes (electroblot)	Leakage	Space samples
		Do not load high level disease
		Load with fresh tips
		Load under buffer
Bands in no DNA control	Contamination	*see* Note 9
Bands in normal DNA	Contamination	*see* Note 9
	Nonspecific hybridization	Increase hybridization temp.
		Increase washing stringency

4. Notes (For General Troubleshooting Notes, *see* Table 2)

1. This provides a standard 1.5-μM magnesium buffer sufficient for 10 100-μL reactions. This is suitable for all the primer systems except TCRγ. With this system, an additional 60 μL of 25 mM MgCl$_2$ is substituted for the equivalent volume of water in each master mix. This gives a final working magnesium concentration of 3 mM.

2. From Table 1, it can be seen that a combination of IgH, Vδ2-Dδ3, and VγI-II and Jγ1/2 are most appropriate for the analysis of B-lineage ALL. Vδ1-Jδ1 and VγI-II and Jγ1/2 are most useful in T-ALL. When ordering oligos, simple desalting is adequate for all PCR, sequencing, and probing applications. We aim to use 1 μg of BM MNC DNA obtained after Ficoll purification and phenol chloroform extraction. More recently a variety of affinity-capture methods have been developed and several provide acceptable alternative methods of DNA extraction. All DNA is screened with an internal Vδ2 control primer pair, which generates a

product of 220 bp (Table 1) to monitor DNA integrity. Peripheral blood is an inferior source of leukemic cells other than at presentation in patients with more than 15×10^9 blasts/L.

3. The method we describe assumes that the required amount of template DNA is suspended in no more than 4 μL of buffer. The use of larger volumes will alter the concentration of the reagents in the reaction adversely. The volume of DNA solution required can be reduced by lyophilizing the sample if necessary. Preparation of reactions on ice ensures consistency.

4. PCR products are resolved by gel electrophoresis. Agarose does not provide adequate resolution of closely spaced, short products. Indeed, using the described primer systems, PCR of polyclonal DNA may show discrete bands following resolution on agarose gels.

5. Probes are extended from a specific hexamer located at the 3' terminus of the sense or antisense primer, by the Klenow fragment of DNA polymerase I. The hexamers used are shown below.

Primer system	Location	Sequence
IgH	FR3A	5'-TACTGT-3'
Vδ2-Dδ3	Dδ3	5'-CGTATC-3'
VγI-II-Jγ1/2	Jγ1/2	5'-GACAAC-3'
Vδ1-Jδ1	Vδ1	5'-AGATTC-3'

6. The potential crosshybridization with common JH primer can be obviated by removal of the primer region by digestion with *Sau* 96 I restriction enzyme prior to labeling *(9)*. This can be performed either directly on whole PCR products or on products previously eluted from gel slices.

7. Although more complex and time consuming, electroblotting is more sensitive and reliable than dot blotting. At times of relative hypo- or hypercellularity, dot blotting can indicate false negative and positive disease, respectively. A fuller discussion of this contrast appears in the legend of Fig. 2 and in Langlands et al., 1994 *(10)*.

8. The optimal slides for this method should be cellular, air dried, and not coverslipped. The presence of stain of any kind does not appear to inhibit amplification. Coverslipped slides can be used if glue can be cleanly removed or dissolved with Histoclear.

   Prior to gene rearrangement PCR, all DNA should be subjected to a control PCR to check for the presence of inhibitors.

9. The spillage of tiny volumes of a PCR reaction (<0.1 μL) can release millions of copies of a PCR product into the laboratory environment *(8)*. This can lead to carry-over of products to subsequent reactions and cause false positive results. The effective prevention of contamination and constant vigilance are the cornerstones of a successful PCR strategy. The following simple precautions are normally all that is required:

   a. DNA extraction and PCR should be performed in an area entirely separate to that used to process PCR products.

   b. Separate laboratory coats, gloves, chemicals, glassware, and pipets should be used.

   c. PCR reactions should be set up in a laminar air-flow hood or on dedicated bench space. Aerosol resistant tips should be used.

   d. Negative controls without template DNA should always be run.

10. To be successful, strategies employing oligonucleotide probes must be based on unequivocal sequence information. We prefer to use solid-phase cycle sequencing with a γ^{33}P-labeled primer. This can be performed directly on the whole PCR reaction if a single clonal product is generated. If multiple products are present, then bands must be excised from PAGE gels prior to sequencing. We find that this method is adequate for more than 90% of clonal products and obviates bidirectional sequencing. Rarely, it is necessary to resort to cloning. In a proportion of patients, direct sequencing cannot be performed owing to close spacing of bands or high polyclonal backgrounds. In such circumstances, cloning is necessary. Various manufacturers produce simple kits facilitating cloning of PCR products. These exploit the 5' adenine overhangs generated by *Taq* polymerase. Efficient ligation of insert is provided by cloning bands eluted from acrylamide and precipitated as above, which removes primer artifacts that readily ligate. A number of recombinant colonies should be screened; if the same sequence occurs twice, this is indicative of a clonal population. Double-stranded recombinant vector can be sequenced according to the linear sequencing protocol described here, although the amount of template can be reduced.

11. The direct sequencing protocol requires PCR products generated with one 5'-biotinylated primer and one nonbiotinylated primer. For optimal results an internal sequencing primer should be used (Table 1). If the sense primer is biotinylated, an antisense sequencing primer should be employed and vice versa. In the absence of biotinylated PCR products, the cycle sequencing protocol is undertaken on DNA eluted from PAGE gels and precipitated as in Section 3.4.1. Proceed directly to the cycle sequencing step (Section 3.5.4).

12. γ^{33}P dATP can be handled on the bench without perspex screens. Alternatively, γ^{32}P dATP can be substituted for γ^{33}P dATP and regular film (e.g., Hyperfilm MP) used. Extra care and screening precautions must be taken.

13. Analysis of logarithmic dilutions provides semiquantitation accurate to within one log. Limiting dilution analysis can provide accurate quantitation but assumes very good quality template DNA and requires exhaustive preparation. Multiple replicate dilutions are required for each time point if this analysis is to be meaningful. The true clinical impact of such an exhaustive approach remains to be seen.

14. It is good practice to perform initial screening and sequence analysis with an inner primer pair. Subsequent residual disease analysis is then performed with an external primer set (*see* Table 1). This reduces the possibility of contamination of remission samples with amplification products from previous reactions. Sequencing also requires an internal primer. This can be achieved by designing a sequencing primer identical to the nonbiotinylated inner primer, but with the two most 5' nucleotides removed (Table 1).

15. It is advisable not to load large amounts of presentation amplification products onto these gels, as the signal generated can obscure the resultant autoradiograph.

It is also imperative to space samples (Figure 2A). Visualization time of bands under UV should be minimized as UV damages DNA.

16. After successful electroblotting, no residual DNA should be detected after staining. Better assessment of transfer is obtained after probing. At this time, we accept transfer of the competed lowest dilution as evidence of low level transfer.

17. Incorporation is assessed by precipitation onto DE-81 paper *(11)* and should be in the region of 30–50%. The use of 10 µL of an end-labeling reaction will provide in excess of the 10^6 dpm/mL prehybridization fluid required. The remainder can be stored for up to 2 wk at –20°C. Unincorporated nucleotides are not removed prior to use.

18. Hybridization is optimally performed in a rotating hybridization oven in glass vessels. It is important to hybridize under stringent conditions. Optimal hybridization temperature is 5–10 degrees below the calculated melting temperature (T_m) of the probe/target duplex. This is calculated according to the following formula:

$$T_m = 81.5 + 16.6(\log10[Na^+]) + 0.41(\%G + C) - 600/L$$

where $[Na^+]$ is the molarity of sodium ions in the buffer (generally $0.5M$), (%G + C) is the percentage G and C content and L the length of the oligonucleotide (20 bases). If patient product probes are used, empirical determination of hybridization temperature is required, but this is usually greater than 65°C.

19. Stringency of washing depends on sodium concentration in the buffer and temperature *(11)*.

References

1. Potter, M. N., Steward, C. G., Maitland, N., and Oakhill, A. (1993) The significance of the detection of minimal residual disease in childhood acute lymphoblastic leukaemia. *Br. J. Haematol.* **83,** 1412–1418.

2. Steward, C. G., Goulden, N. J., Katz, F., Baines, D., Martin, P. G., Langlands, K., Potter, M. N., Chessells, J. M., and Oakhill, A. (1994) A polymerase chain reaction study of the stability of immunoglobulin heavy chain and T-cell receptor d gene rearrangements between presentation and relapse of childhood B-lineage acute lymphoblastic leukemia. *Blood* **83,** 1355–1362.

3. Steward, C. G., Goulden, N. J., Potter, M. N., and Oakhill A. (1993) The use of the polymerase chain reaction to detect minimal residual disease in childhood acute lymphoblastic leukaemia. *Eur. J. Cancer* **8,** 1192–1198.

4. Yamada, M., Hudson, S., Tournay, O., Bittenbender, S., Shane, S. S., Lange, B., Tsujimoto, Y., Caton, A. J., and Rovera, G. (1989) Detection of minimal disease in haemopoetic malignancies of the B-cell lineage by using third-complementarity-determining region (CDR-III)-specific probes. *Proc. Natl. Acad. Sci. USA* **86,** 5123–5127.

5. Yokota, S., Hansen-Hagge, T. E., Ludwig, W. D., Reiter, A., Raghavachar, A., Kleihauer, E., and Bartram, C. R. (1991) Use of polymerase chain reactions to monitor minimal residual disease in acute lymphoblastic leukaemia patients. *Blood* **77,** 331–339.

6. Brisco, M. J., Tan, L. W., Osborn, A. M., and Morley, A. A. (1990) Development of a highly sensitive assay, based on the polymerase chain reaction, for rare B-lymphocyte clones in a polyclonal population. *Br. J. Haematol.* **75,** 163–167.
7. Murray, V. (1989) Improved double-stranded DNA sequencing using the linear polymerase chain reaction. *Nucleic Acids Res.* **17,** 8889.
8. Kwok, S. and Higuchi, R. (1989) Avoiding false positives with PCR. *Nature* **339,** 237–238.
9. Nizet, Y., Van Daele, S., Lewalle, P., Vaerman, J. L., Philippe, M., Vermylen, C., Cornu, G., Ferrant, A., Michaux, J. L., and Martiat, P. (1994) Long-term follow-up of residual disease in acute lymphoblastic leukemia patients in complete remission using clonogenic IgH probes and the polymerase chain reaction. *Blood* **82,** 1618–1625.
10. Langlands, K., Goulden, N. J., Steward, C. G., Potter, M. N., Cornish, J. M., and Oakhill, A. (1994) False positive residual disease assessment post-bone marrow transplant in acute lymphoblastic leukaemia. *Blood* **84,** 1352,1353 (letter).
11. Sambrook, J., Fritch, E. F., and Maniatis, T. (1989) *Molecular Cloning: A Laboratory Manual,* 2nd ed., Cold Spring Harbor Laboratory, Cold Spring Harbor, NY.

2

Detection of BCR-ABL
in Hematological Malignancies by RT-PCR

Nicholas C. P. Cross

1. Introduction

The presence of a novel, minute chromosome in the cells of patients with chronic myeloid leukemia (CML) was first described in 1960 by Nowell and Hungerford (1). The Philadelphia (Ph) chromosome, as it became known, was shown subsequently by banding techniques to result from a reciprocal translocation between the long arms of chromosomes 9 and 22 t(9;22) (q34;q11) (2). Molecular studies demonstrated that the translocation disrupted the normal ABL and BCR genes on chromosomes 9 and 22, respectively, giving rise to a chimeric BCR-ABL gene encoding a fusion protein with transforming ability (3). The reciprocal ABL-BCR product is also transcriptionally active in the majority of cases (4,5).

The standard Ph chromosome is found in ~90% of cases of CML and cytogenetic variants account for a further 5%. Of the remaining 5%, roughly half show a BCR-ABL fusion mRNA by PCR, whereas the rest are considered to be Ph-negative, BCR-ABL-negative CML (6). Occasional patients initially diagnosed as having essential thrombocythemia (ET) or agnogenic myeloid metaplasia (AMM) are also Ph-positive. The Ph chromosome is also the single most common chromosomal abnormality in acute lymphoblastic leukemia (ALL) in which roughly 5% of children and 20% or more of adults are positive. Furthermore, about 1% of acute myeloid leukemias (AML) are Ph-positive (6). Although the translocation breakpoints are widely dispersed, especially within the very large ABL first intron (7), after splicing of the primary transcript the vast majority of CML patients have breakpoints that result in a fusion mRNA in which either BCR exon b2 or b3 is fused to ABL exon a2 (b2a2 or b3a2 transcripts). Both transcripts give rise to a 210-kDa BCR-ABL protein (3).

From: *Methods in Molecular Medicine, Molecular Diagnosis of Cancer*
Edited by: F. E. Cotter Humana Press Inc., Totowa, NJ

Approximately 70% of Ph-positive ALL cases have breakpoints that result in the fusion of BCR exon e1 to ABL exon a2 (e1a2 transcript), which is translated into the smaller 190-kDa BCR-ABL protein; the remaining 30% have a 210-kDa BCR-ABL product indistinguishable from that found in CML *(8)*.

The polymerase chain reaction (PCR) is a rapid and powerful method for detection of specific sequences and has been used to amplify to BCR-ABL cDNA after reverse transcription of the mRNA. PCR efficiently detects BCR-ABL in BCR-rearranged, Ph negative patients and may also be used to detect minimal residual disease up to a sensitivity of a single leukemia cell in a background of 10^5–10^6 normal cells *(9–12)*. The techniques thus are of use diagnostically and for monitoring response to therapy.

Conditions are presented here for the unambiguous and rapid determination of the presence or absence of BCR-ABL transcripts in patient samples. For diagnostic samples, randomly primed cDNA is synthesized from leukocyte RNA and amplified in a single reaction containing four oligonucleotide primers *(13)*. Different size products are generated from the various BCR-ABL transcripts that are readily and unambiguously distinguishable after agarose gel electrophoresis without the need for either nested PCR or hybridization. BCR-ABL negative samples generate a specific BCR amplification product that serves as a control for satisfactory cDNA. For remission samples a two-step, nested, PCR for either p210 or p190 BCR-ABL transcripts is described *(11)* and also a competitive PCR assay for quantification of residual disease *(14)*.

2. Materials

2.1. RT-PCR

1. Red cell lysis buffer (RCLB): $0.155M$ NH_4Cl, 10 mM $KHCO_3$, 0.1 mM EDTA made to pH 7.4 at 0°C with $2M$ HCL (do not autoclave).
2. Phosphate-buffered saline (PBS): Made up from stock tablets (Oxoid, Basingstoke, UK) and autoclaved.
3. $1M$ citrate pH 7.0: Neutralize $1M$ trisodium citrate with $1M$ citric acid.
4. GTC: $4M$ Guanidinium thiocyanate (Fluka, Buchs, Switzerland), 5 mM EDTA, 25 mM citrate, pH 7.0, 0.5% sarcosyl (BDH, Poole, UK). Do not autoclave but make up using DEPC-treated $1M$ citrate, pH 7.0, $0.5M$ EDTA, pH 8.0 and H_2O. Add 7.1 μL β-mercaptoethanol/mL of GTC immediately before use.
5. CsCl cushion: $5.7M$ CsCl, 1 mM EDTA, 25 mM citrate, pH 7.0. Treat with DEPC (*see* Note 1).
6. TES: 10 mM Tris-HCl, pH 7.5, 10 mM EDTA, 0.1% SDS made up with DEPC-treated water and $0.5M$ EDTA, pH 8.0.
7. Sodium acetate (NaOAc): $3M$ brought to pH 5.2, or $2M$ brought to pH 4.0, with glacial acetic acid and treated with DEPC.

8. 70% ethanol made up with DEPC-treated water.
9. Carrier RNA: *E. coli* tRNA (Sigma, St. Louis, MO) or *E. coli* rRNA (Boehringer Mannheim, Mannheim, Germany) made up to 1 mg/mL with DEPC-treated water.
10. Random hexamer primers: 50 U pdN$_6$ (Pharmacia, Uppsala, Sweden) dissolved in 539 µL DEPC-treated water plus 21 µL 0.5M KCl. Final concentration = 5 mg/mL.
11. 5X RT buffer: 0.25M Tris-HCl, pH 8.3, 0.375 mM KCl, 15 mM MgCl$_2$. Supplied with M-MLV reverse transcriptase (Gibco-BRL, Gaithersburg, MD) along with 0.1M dithiothreitol (DTT).
12. 25 mM dNTP stock: Mix an equal volume of ultrapure 100 mM dATP, dCTP, dGTP, and dTTP (Pharmacia). Store at –70°C.
13. cDNA mix (per mL): Mix 428 µL of 5X RT buffer, 21.5 µL of 0.1M DTT, 85.5 µL of 25 mM dNTPs, 45 µL of 5 mg/mL random hexamers and 420 µL of DEPC-treated water.
14. 10X *Taq* Pol buffer: 100 mM Tris-HCl, pH 8.3, 500 mM KCl (usually supplied with the enzyme along with 50 mM MgCl$_2$).
15. Oligonucleotide primers: All primers were diluted to 1 mg/mL before making up the mixes that follow.
16. Multiplex PCR mix (per mL): Mix 120 µL of 10X *Taq* Pol buffer, 9.6 µL of 25 mM dNTPs, 45 µL of 50 mM MgCl$_2$, 5.6 µL of primer CA3-, 5.3 µL of primer C5e-, 5 µL of primer B2B, 4.4 µL of primer BCR-C, and 805 µL of water.
17. p210 first step mix (per mL): Mix 125 µL of 10X *Taq* Pol buffer, 10 µL of 25 mM dNTPs, 62.5 µL of 50 mM MgCl$_2$, 5.2 µL of primer NB1+, 5.4 µL of primer ABL3-, and 792 µL of water.
18. p210 second step mix (per mL): Mix 100 µL of 10X *Taq* Pol buffer, 8 µL of 25 mM dNTPs, 35 µL of 50 mM MgCl$_2$, 4.6 µL of primer CA3-, 3.6 µL of primer B2A, and 849 µL of water.
19. p190 first step mix (per mL): Mix 125 µL of 10X *Taq* Pol buffer, 10 µL of 25 mM dNTPs, 45 µL of 50 mM MgCl$_2$, 4.5 µL of primer BCR-B, 5.4 µL of primer ABL3-, and 810 µL of water.
20. p190 second step mix (per mL): Mix 125 µL of 10X *Taq* Pol buffer, 10 µL of 25 mM dNTPs, 43 µL of 50 mM MgCl$_2$, 4.6 µL of primer CA3-, 3.6 µL of primer BCR1+, and 813 µL of water.
21. Competitor constructs: We have used plasmids pBKλ5 and p190-C5 *(14,18)* to quantify p210 and p190 BCR-ABL transcripts, respectively. For use, the plasmids are linearized with either *Bam*HI (p210) or *Eco*RI (p190) and then diluted in 1 mM Tris-HCl, pH 8.0, 0.1 mM EDTA, 50 µg/mL *E. coli* tRNA. Dilutions are made in the range from 10^7–10 mol/2.5 µL with steps at every half order of magnitude on a logarithmic scale, i.e., 10^7, 3.2×10^6, 10^6, and so on.

The cDNA mix and all of the PCR mixes should be divided into small, single use aliquots and kept at –70°C. Specific manufacturers have been indicated for some products that we have found to work well, however, products from other sources may, of course, be substituted.

2.2. Oligonucleotide Primers

BCR1+	5' GAACTCGCAACAGTCCTTCGAC 3'
BCR-B	5' CCCCCGGAGTTTTGAGGATTGC 3'
BCR-C	5' ACCGCATGTTCCGGGACAAAAG 3'
B2B	5' ACAGaATTCCGCTGACCATCAATAAG 3'
C5e-	5' ataggaTCCTTTGCAACCGGGTCTGAA 3'
NB1+	5' GAGCGTGCAGAGTGGAGGGAGAACA 3'
ABL3-	5' GGTACCAGGAGTGTTTCTCCAGACTG 3'
B2A	5' TTCAGAAGCTTCTCCCTGACAT 3'
CA3-	5' TGTTGACTGGCGTGATGTAGTTGCTTGG 3'

Lower case letters denote bases that were changed from the natural sequence in order to introduce restriction enzyme sites. These sites are not relevant to the applications described here. Positions of the primers are shown on Fig. 1.

3. Methods

3.1. Sample Preparation (see Note 1)

1. Spin blood or marrow sample at 1500 rpm for 10 min (*see* Notes 2–5).
2. Working from the top, carefully remove 80% of the plasma and discard. Take the rest of the plasma (buffy coat) down to approx 1/2 cm into the red cells into a 50-mL tube.
3. Fill tube with ice-cold RCLB. Leave on ice for 10 min with intermittent shaking.
4. Spin down leukocytes 10 min, 1500 rpm. If pellet is very red, repeat RCLB lysis.
5. Wash pellet once with 20 mL PBS and spin down again.
6. For RNA extraction method A, add 2.5 mL GTC containing 0.37 g/mL CsCl (freshly added) to the cell pellet (maximum 2×10^8 cells). Using a syringe, rapidly homogenize and shear the DNA by passing several times through a needle. If $<10^7$ cells, add 50 µg *E. coli* rRNA.
7. For RNA extraction method B, resuspend cells and transfer a maximum of 2×10^7 into a microfuge tube. After pelleting the cells, remove PBS, dislodge the pellet by vortexing briefly, add 500 µL GTC (without CsCl) and vortex for 10 s. If $<10^6$ cells, add 5 µg *E. coli* tRNA.
8. Store GTC lysates at 4°C for up to 1 wk, or long-term at –20°C.

3.2. RNA Extraction (see Note 6)

3.2.1. Method A (Modified from ref. 15)

1. Put 1 mL CsCl cushion into a Beckman (Fullerton, CA) conical ultracentrifuge tube and layer the GTC lysate carefully on top. Always include at least one blank (*see* Note 7) at this stage (50 µg *E. coli* rRNA in GTC).
2. Spin 40,000g for 16 h in an SW55, or other swingout rotor at 20°C.
3. Remove approx 3 mL of the liquid carefully from the top using a disposable sterile plastic pipet (*see* Note 8).
4. Pour off the remaining liquid and invert the tube to drain for 5 min.
5. Dry sides of tube with a sterile tissue.

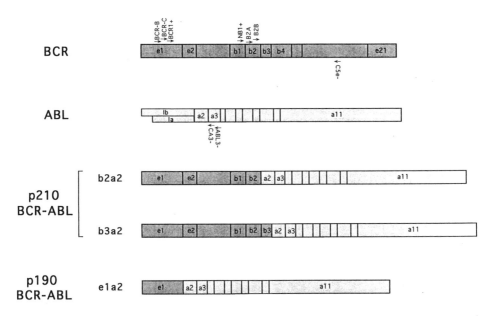

Fig. 1. Schematic representation of the normal BCR gene, the normal ABL gene and the three BCR-ABL derivatives (not to scale). The approximate positions of the oligonucleotide primers are indicated.

6. Add 250 µL TES to (invisible) pellet. Mix up and down with a pipet, leave for 10 min, mix up and down again, and transfer to a microfuge tube.
7. Add 25 µL 3*M* NaOAc pH 5.2 and 750 µL absolute ethanol and leave at −20°C for at least 2 h.
8. Spin 10 min at top speed. Take off all liquid and wash pellet with 1 mL 80% ethanol.
9. Take off all liquid and let pellet air dry for 10 min.
10. Dissolve the RNA in DEPC-treated water (e.g., 40 µL). Dilute an aliquot for spectrophotometric determination of concentration (1 OD U at 260 nm = 40 µg/mL). Usually 20 mL peripheral blood yields 5–40 µg RNA.

3.2.2. Method B (AGCP Method Modified from ref. 16)

1. Add 50 µL 2*M* NaOAc pH 4.0 to 500 µL GTC lysate. Always include at least one blank.
2. Add 500 µL unneutralized water-saturated phenol and 100 µL chloroform. Vortex for 10 s.
3. Cool on ice 20 min and then spin at top speed 20 min at 4°C.
4. Take top layer into new tube. Do not disturb the interface and leave 50–100 µL behind. If the phases have not separated well, add another 50 µL of chloroform, vortex, and spin again.

5. Add equal volume of propan-2-ol (isopropanol), mix, and leave at –20°C for at least 1 h.
6. Spin 15 min at 4°C, remove all supernatant, and wash the RNA pellet with 1 mL 80% ethanol.
7. Respin, take off all the liquid, and let the pellet air dry for 10 min.
8. Dissolve the RNA in DEPC-treated water (e.g., 40 μL).

3.2. cDNA Synthesis

1. Take, per reaction, 20 μL of cDNA mix and add 300 U M-MLV reverse transcriptase and 30 U RNasin.
2. Heat 19 μL RNA (maximum 20 μg) to 65°C for 5 min and place on ice. Introduce another negative control (water blank) at this stage.
3. Add 21 μL of cDNA mix to RNA (*see* Notes 9 and 10). Place at 37°C for 2 h. Store remaining RNA at –70°C.
4. Terminate reaction by heating to 65°C for 10 min. Store cDNA at –20°C.

3.3. Multiplex PCR (see Note 11)

1. Take, per reaction, 21 μL multiplex PCR mix and add 0.75 U *Taq* polymerase.
2. Add 4 μL of cDNA (*see* Note 9) and one drop of mineral oil.
3. Amplify for 30–35 cycles at 96°C 30 s, 60°C 50 s, 72°C 1 min, followed by a 10 min extension at 72°C (*see* Note 12).
4. Electrophorese 10 μL of the reaction on a 1.5% agarose gel containing 0.2 μg/mL ethidium bromide. Bands should be as follows: 808 bp, normal BCR (B2B to C5e-); 481 bp, e1a2 (BCR-C to CA3-); 385 bp and/or 310 bp, b3a2 and b2a2, respectively (B2B to CA3-). An amplified product from the BCR gene is the only band detected in those patients who are BCR-ABL-negative (Fig. 2). The sole presence of this band indicates that the quality of the RNA and efficiency of cDNA synthesis were good; thus the patient confidently can be considered to be negative for BCR-ABL. Absence of any band indicates failure of the procedure (*see* Notes 13–16).

3.4. Nested PCR (see Notes 11 and 17)

1. Take, per reaction, 20 μL first step PCR (either p210 or p190) mix, and add 0.75 U *Taq* polymerase.
2. Add 5 μL of cDNA and one drop of mineral oil. Include a further negative control.
3. Amplify for 30 cycles at 96°C 30 s, 68°C 25 s, 72°C 1 min (for p210), or at 96°C 30 s, 64°C 50 s, 72°C 1 min (for p190), followed by a 10-min extension at 72°C.
4. Take, per reaction, 19 μL appropriate second step mix and add 0.75 U *Taq* polymerase.
5. Add 1 μL of the first step reaction and one drop of mineral oil.
6. Amplify for 30 cycles at 96°C 30 s, 64°C 50 s, 72°C 1 min, followed by a 10 min extension at 72°C (for either p210 or p190).
7. Electrophorese 10 μL of the second step reaction on a 1.5% agarose gel containing 0.2 μg/mL ethidium bromide. Bands should be 458 bp (b3a2), 383 bp (b2a2), or 444 bp (e1a2).

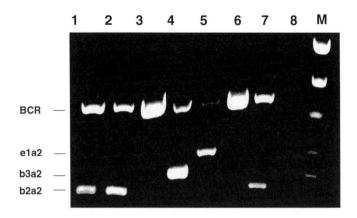

Fig. 2. Multiplex PCR. Lanes 1 and 2: Ph-positive CML, both with b2a2 BCR-ABL; lane 3: Ph-negative, BCR-ABL-negative CML; lane 4: Ph negative b3a2 BCR-ABL positive CML; lanes 5 and 7: Ph-positive ALL with e1a2 and b2a2 BCR-ABL respectively; lane 6: Ph-negative, BCR-ABL-negative ALL, lane 8: negative control; lane M: pEMBL/*Taq*1 markers.

3.5. Competitive (Quantitative) PCR (14)

1. As nested PCR except that 2.5 μL of cDNA plus 2.5 μL competitor are used as templates for the first step PCR; and 1 μL of the first step reaction is diluted into 200 μL H$_2$O and 1 μL of this dilution used to seed the second step PCR. A series of reactions are performed, initially adding competitor at every order of magnitude and then homing in to the equivalence point at every half order of magnitude.
2. After electrophoresis, the competitor bands are distinguishable from the sample BCR-ABL by size. The p210 competitor gives a band at 559 bp and the p190 competitor at 578 bp.
3. The number of BCR-ABL transcripts in the specimen is determined by the number of competitor molecules that are added, or would have to be added, to give competitor and BCR-ABL bands of equal intensity. This may be estimated by eye or by densitometry. Compensation for the difference in size between the bands is made by multiplying the number of competitor molecules added at the equivalence point by 1.2 (b3a2), 1.5 (b2a2), or 1.3 (e1a2). Knowing the amount of RNA used to make the cDNA, this number can be converted to the number of BCR-ABL transcripts/μg RNA (*see* Notes 18 and 19).

4. Notes

1. The problem of contamination in PCR analysis cannot be overemphasized. Although it is possible to perform PCR with few precautions for many months without spurious results, once contamination does arise it may be surprisingly difficult to eliminate. Multiple negative controls should always be performed and results discarded if any negative controls are positive. To avoid contamination,

PCR products must be kept separate from all of the previous steps, i.e., sample and reagent preparation, RNA extraction, cDNA synthesis, and PCR setup. The simplest, and most effective, way to do this is to always electrophorese the reaction products in a second laboratory using a different set of pipets. Plasmids or other clones may also be a serious source of contamination if they harbor the relevant sequences; such clones should always be manipulated in a different laboratory from where the PCRs are set up. The use of plugged (aerosol-resistant) pipet tips and laminar flow hood may help to minimize contamination. We have found it helpful to designate all stock solutions and chemicals for PCR use only, and to make up large batches of cDNA synthesis and PCR reagents in single-use aliquots; this has the added advantage of improving the reproducibility of the assay.

Care must be taken in the preparation and manipulation of RNA in order to prevent degradation by ubiquitous ribonucleases (RNase). Gloves should always be worn and changed frequently. Aqueous solutions that do not contain Tris or SDS should be treated by addition of diethylpyrocarbonate (DEPC) to 0.1%, incubation for 2 h at 37°C followed by autoclaving. It is not usually necessary to treat pipet tips and microfuge tubes as long as they are sterile and only handled using gloves.

2. Either blood or bone marrow may be used for diagnostic samples. For residual disease studies, blood and marrow are of equal sensitivity for CML *(17)*, whereas marrow is preferred for ALL *(18)*.

3. Red cells may also be removed by isolating mononuclear cells after centrifugation over Lymphoprep, according to the manufacturer's instructions.

4. Samples are usually 20 mL peripheral blood or 2 mL bone marrow, but diagnostic samples may be as little as 25 µL. Generally, it is important to remove the bulk of the red cells but whole blood or marrow may be lysed directly provided the sample volume does not exceed 5% of the volume of GTC.

5. The best way to store samples is as lysates in GTC at –20°C in which they are stable for months or even years. Extracted RNA is nearly always of inferior quality if cryopreserved cells or frozen cell pellets are used rather than fresh material.

6. We find RNA extraction method A gives the most reliable results and is more appropriate for residual disease studies since it is necessary to use larger samples in order to achieve the maximum sensitivity. Method B has the advantage that an ultracentrifuge is not required and usually is the method of choice when a large number of samples need to be processed.

7. Although it is important to always include multiple negative controls to monitor for contamination, it is also important to include positive controls to check for efficiency and sensitivity, particularly for residual disease studies. Convenient positive controls are RNA extracted from cell lines, e.g., b3a2, K562 *(19)*; b2a2, BV173 *(20)*; e1a2, SD1 *(21)*.

8. The supernatant contains the DNA which, if sufficient cells are processed, forms an easily identifiable a viscous layer. To recover the DNA, dilute the viscous layer with 4 vol H_2O, extract twice with an equal volume of 1:1 neutralized phenol/chloroform and precipitate with 2 vol of ethanol.

9. The final concentrations of reagents in the reverse transcription reaction are: 50 mM Tris-HCl, pH 8.3, 75 mM KCl, 3 mM MgCl$_2$, 1 mM DTT, 120 μg/mL random hexamers, 1.4 × 10^4 U/mL M-MLV reverse transcriptase, 1400 U/mL RNasin. The final concentrations in the PCR are: 10 mM Tris-HCl, pH 8.3, 50 mM KCl, 1.5–2.5 mM MgCl$_2$ 0.5 μM primers, 0.2 mM each of dATP, dGTP, dCTP, and dTTP, 30 U/mL *Taq* polymerase.

10. Too much cDNA inhibits the amplification efficiency. If a background smear, or weak/absent bands are obtained, try reducing the amount of cDNA used to seed the PCR.

11. The multiplex PCR easily should be able to detect BCR-ABL when chronic phase CML blood is diluted into normal blood at a ratio of 1:100. It should not be necessary to use nested PCR to detect BCR-ABL in samples at diagnosis. Nested PCR should routinely detect a single leukemia cell in a background of 10^5–10^6 normal cells and therefore is used to detect residual disease in patients who are in cytogenetic remission. This great sensitivity, however, can lead to serious problems with contamination.

12. The precise cycling conditions need to be optimized for each thermocycler and therefore these parameters are given as a guide only. Common causes of failure are lack of primer binding because the annealing temperature is too high, or inefficient strand separation owing to the denaturing temperature being too low.

13. PCRs may fail if the Mg^{2+} concentration is too low and therefore the MgCl$_2$ concentrations given here are slightly greater than in previous recipes. Other common reasons for failure of amplification are poor quality cDNA or that either *Taq* polymerase or nucleotides have gone off.

14. Specificity is often improved by "hot-start" PCR in which the *Taq* polymerase is added only after once the tubes have reached the denaturation temperature. We have found that usually the same specificity can be achieved by allowing the thermocycler to heat up to 96°C before putting in the reaction tubes.

15. In those patients expressing BCR-ABL, the BCR band derived from the normal allele is sometimes not visible. This is not due to a failure of BCR expression in these patients, since BCR is effectively amplified if primers B2B and C5e- are used on their own; presumably the BCR-ABL amplification product effectively out competes or suppresses the BCR product under the reaction conditions described. Occasionally an additional band is seen at about 2.3 kb. This results from amplification of the normal BCR allele with primers BCR-C and C5e-.

16. Other genes may be amplified in a separate reaction to control for adequate cDNA synthesis. However, since RNA preparations always contain variable amounts of contaminating genomic DNA, it is crucial to confirm that primers used for the control gene do not generate an amplification product from genomic DNA that may be confused with that from cDNA. It is also important to use a control gene that is expressed at a similar level to the target gene. For example, β-actin should not be used as a control for RT-PCR since this gene is expressed at a much higher level than BCR-ABL and furthermore the genome contains multiple β-actin pseudogenes *(22,23)*.

17. The simple detection or nondetection of BCR-ABL mRNA by nested PCR in remission samples is of limited value in the clinical management of individual patients *(12)*. In response to this, we and others developed a competitive PCR assay to quantitate BCR-ABL transcripts and showed that rising levels of the fusion gene mRNA can be observed several months prior to cytogenetic detection of relapse *(14,24)*. Furthermore such evidence of early relapse may be used to initiate effective therapy in the form of donor lymphocyte transfusion *(25)*.

18. Chronic phase CML samples should have about 2×10^5–10^6 BCR-ABL transcripts/µg RNA. Levels in diagnostic ALL samples may be somewhat higher. Patients who are in cytogenetic remission generally have $<5 \times 10^3$ BCR-ABL transcripts/µg RNA *(14)*.

19. Extensive controls are needed to monitor the reproducibility of competitive PCR. A range of dilutions of positive RNAs and cDNA should be stored and tested frequently. Although the competitive PCR described here controls effectively for variations in PCR amplification efficiency, it does not control for the quality of the RNA, the efficiency of the cDNA synthesis or the quantity of RNA (if the RNA is contaminated with DNA or the amount of RNA is small, then large errors may be introduced by spectrophotometric determination of concentration). Probably the most robust way to control for all these parameters is to quantify BCR-ABL relative to an internal control gene. We are exploring the use of ABL and other genes as internal controls for competitive PCR *(18)*.

References

1. Nowell, P. C. and Hungerford, D. A. (1960) A minute chromosome in chronic granulocytic leukemia. *Science* **132,** 1497.
2. Rowley, J. D. (1973) A new consistent chromosomal abnormality in chronic myelogenous leukaemia identified by quinacrine fluorescence and Giemsa staining. *Nature* **243,** 290–293.
3. Groffen, J. and Heisterkamp, N. (1987) The BCR/ABL hybrid gene. *Baillieres Clin. Haematol.* **1,** 983–999.
4. Melo, J. V., Gordon, D. E., Cross, N. C. P., and Goldman, J. M. (1993) The ABL-BCR fusion gene is expressed in chronic myeloid leukemia. *Blood* **81,** 158–165.
5. Melo, J. V., Gordon, D. E., Tuszynski, A., Dhut, S., Young, B. D., and Goldman, J. M. (1993) Expression of the ABL-BCR fusion gene in Philadelphia-positive acute lymphoblastic leukemia. *Blood* **81,** 2488–2491.
6. Hagemeijer, A. (1987) Chromosome abnormalities in CML. *Baillieres Clin. Haematol.* **1,** 963–981.
7. Bernards, A., Rubin, C. M., Westbrook, C. A., Paskind, M., and Baltimore, D. (1987) The first intron in the human c-abl gene is at least 200kb long and is a target for translocations in chronic myelogenous leukemia. *Mol. Cell. Biol.* **7,** 3231–3236.
8. Maurer, J., Janssen, J. W. G., Thiel, E., van Denderen, J., Ludwig, W. D., Aydemir, U., Heinze, B., Fonatsch, C., Harbott, J., Reiter, A., Riehm, H., Hoelzer, D., and Bartram, C. R. (1991) Detection of chimeric BCR-ABL genes in acute lymphoblastic leukaemia by the polymerase chain reaction. *Lancet* **337,** 1055–1058.

9. Kawasaki, E. S., Clark, S. S., Coyne, M. Y., Smith, S. D., Champlin, R., Witte, O. N., and McCormick, F. P. (1988) Diagnosis of chronic myeloid and acute lymphocytic leukemias by detection of leukemia-specific mRNA sequences amplified in vitro. *Proc. Natl. Acad. Sci. USA* **85**, 5698–5702.

10. Hughes, T. P., Morgan, G. J., Martiat, P., and Goldman, J. M. (1991) Detection of residual leukemia after bone marrow transplant for chronic myeloid leukemia: role of polymerase chain reaction in predicting relapse. *Blood* **77**, 874–878.

11. Cross, N. C. P., Hughes, T. P., Feng, L., O'Shea, P., Bungey, J., Marks, D. I., Ferrant, A., Martiat, P., and Goldman, J. M. (1993) Minimal residual disease after allogeneic bone marrow transplantation for chronic myeloid leukaemia in first chronic phase: correlations with acute graft-versus-host disease and relapse. *Br. J. Haematol.* **84**, 67–74.

12. Miyamura, K., Barrett, A. J., Kodera, Y., and Saito, H. (1994) Minimal residual disease after bone marrow transplantation for chronic myelogenous leukemia and implications for graft-versus-leukemia effect: a review of recent results. *Bone Marrow Transplantation* **14**, 201–209.

13. Cross, N. C. P., Melo, J. V., Lin, F., and Goldman, J. M. (1994) An optimised multiplex polymerase chain reaction for detection of BCR-ABL fusion mRNAs in hematological disorders. *Leukemia* **8**, 186–189.

14. Cross, N. C. P., Lin, F., Chase, A., Bungey, J., and Hughes, T. P., Goldman, J. M. (1993) Competitive polymerase chain reaction to estimate the number of BCR-ABL transcripts in chronic myeloid leukemia patients after bone marrow transplantation. *Blood* **82**, 1929–1936.

15. Glisin, V., Crkvenjakov, R., and Byus, C. (1974) Ribonucleic acid isolated by cesium chloride centrifugation. *Biochemistry* **13**, 2633–2639.

16. Chomczynski, P. and Sacchi, N. (1987) Single-step method of RNA isolation by acid guanidinium thiocyanate-phenol-chloroform extraction. *Anal. Biochem.* **162**, 156–159.

17. Lin, F., Goldman, J. M., and Cross, N. C. P. (1994) A comparison of the sensitivity of blood and bone marrow for the detection of minimal residual disease in chronic myeloid leukaemia. *Br. J. Haematol.* **86**, 683–685.

18. van Rhee, F., Marks, D. I., Lin, F., Szydlo, R., Hochhans, A., Treleaven, J., Delord, C., Cross, N. C. P., and Goldman, J. M. (1995) Quantification of residual disease in Philadelphia-positive acute lymphoblastic leukemia—comparison of blood and bone marrow. *Leukemia* **9**, 329–335.

19. Lozzio, C. B. and Lozzio, B. B. (1975) Human chronic myelogenous leukemia cell line with positive Philadelphia chromosome. *Blood* **45**, 321–334.

20. Pegoraro, L., Matera, L., Ritz, J., Levis, A., Palumbo, A., and Biagini, G. (1983) Establishment of a Ph-positive cell line (BV173). *J. Natl. Cancer Inst.* **70**, 447–453.

21. Dhut, S., Gibbons, B., Chaplin, T., and Young, B. D. (1991) Establishment of a lymphoblastoid cell line, SD-1, expressing the p190 bcr-abl chimaeric protein. *Leukemia* **5**, 49–55.

22. Cross, N. C. P., Lin, F., and Goldman, J. M. (1994) Appropriate controls for reverse transcription polymerase chain reaction (RT-PCR). *Br. J. Haematol.* **87**, 218.

23. Taylor, J. J. and Heasman, P. A. (1994) Control genes for reverse transcriptase/polymerase chain reaction (RT-PCR). *Br. J. Haematol.* **86,** 444–445.
24. Lion, T., Henn, T., Gaiger, A., Kalhs, P., and Gadner, H. (1993) Early detection of relapse after bone marrow transplantation in patients with chronic myelogenous leukaemia. *Lancet* **341,** 275–276.
25. van Rhee, F., Lin, F., Cullis, J. O., Spencer, A., Cross, N. C. P., Chase, A., Garicochea, B., Bungey, J., Barrett, J. A., Goldman, and J. M. (1994) Relapse of chronic myeloid leukemia after allogeneic bone marrow transplant: the case for giving donor leukocyte transfusions before the onset of hematologic relapse. *Blood* **83,** 3377–3383.

3

Molecular Diagnosis of Acute Myeloid Leukemia with Maturation, FAB-Type M2

Ewald J. B. M. Mensink and Louis T. F. van de Locht

1. Introduction

Nonrandom chromosome abnormalities frequently are seen in particular subtypes of human leukemia and lymphoma. These abnormalities are considered to be involved in the neoplastic transformation and in tumor progression. The translocation (8;21) (q22;q22) is consistently associated with acute myeloid leukemia with maturation (French-American-British classification subtype M2; AML-M2). It accounts for 40% of pediatric type AML-M2. Molecular cloning of the chromosome 8–21 translocation breakpoint showed clustering on chromosome 21 within a limited region in the AML1 gene and on chromosome 8 within a limited region in the ETO gene (Eight Twenty One) also called MTG8 (Myeloid Translocation Gene on chromosome 8) *(1–7)*. The t(8;21) results in a chimerical AML1/ETO gene on the der(8) chromosome. Rearrangement of AML1 was also detected in a patient with 8q- and only one chromosome 21, but without 21q+. This indicates that the molecular events on the der(8) chromosome leading to the chimerical AML1/ETO gene are more important than the events on the reciprocal 21q+ chromosome *(8)*.

The role of the chimerical AML1/ETO protein in oncogenesis is as yet unknown. The ETO gene is not normally expressed in the hematopoietic system. Expression of a 5.5 kb ETO mRNA was found in the lung *(9)*. Based upon the protein structure, the AML1 protein was proposed to be a transcription factor *(5)*. The central part of the AML1 protein contains a region of homology to the *runt* segmentation gene of *Drosophila (1)*. The AML1 gene is also involved in the t(3;21) occurring in therapy-related leukemia and in chronic myeloid leukemia in blast crisis *(10,11)*. In both types of translocation, this *runt* domain is retained in the chimerical protein. This domain was shown to be important for sequence-specific DNA binding and protein–protein interactions *(12)*.

From: *Methods in Molecular Medicine, Molecular Diagnosis of Cancer*
Edited by: F. E. Cotter Humana Press Inc., Totowa, NJ

Southern blotting and polymerase chain reaction (PCR) can be used as useful tools for the diagnosis and monitoring of the disease. They could prove to be useful in assessing residual leukemia after chemotherapy and be important in deciding further treatment.

2. Materials

As a positive control in the Southern blotting and RT-PCR genomic DNA and mRNA derived from cell line Kasumi-1 can be used. This cell line carries the t(8;21) and has characteristics of myeloid and macrophage lineages *(13)*. It can be obtained from the European Collection of Animal Cell Cultures (Salisbury, UK; ref. no. 8550). As a negative control, DNA and mRNA of peripheral blood mononuclear cells of healthy individuals can be used (*see* Note 1). p52

2.1. Small-Scale RNA Isolation

All solutions and glassware should be DEPC treated to remove RNases.

1. Guanidinium-isothiocyanate solution (GITC): $4M$ guanidinium-isothiocyanate, 25 mM sodium citrate pH 7, 0.5% *N*-lauroyl sarcosine, and 0.1M β-mercaptoethanol.
2. 10 mg/mL Yeast t-RNA (Boehringer/Mannheim, Mannheim Germany).
3. $2M$ Sodium acetate, pH 4.0.
4. Water-saturated phenol.
5. Chloroform.
6. Isoamylalcohol.
7. Isopropanol.
8. DEPC-treated dH_2O.

2.2. cDNA Synthesis

1. 200 U/μL Mo-MLV Reverse transcriptase (Gibco/BRL, Gaithersburg, MD).
2. 5X Reverse transcriptase buffer: 250 mM Tris-HCl, pH 8.3, 375 mM KCl, 15 mM MgCl$_2$.
3. 100 mM DTT.
4. dNTP mixture of 25 mM of each nucleotide (Pharmacia, Uppsala, Sweden).
5. 100 pmol/μL Random hexamers (Boehringer/Mannheim).
6. 40 U/μL RNasin RNase inhibitor (Promega, Madison, WI).

2.3. Polymerase Chain Reaction

1. 10X PCR buffer: 200 mM Tris-HCl, pH 8.3, 500 mM KCl, 15 mM MgCl$_2$, 0.01% gelatin.
2. 5 U/μL *Taq* Polymerase (Gibco/BRL).
3. 10 pmol/μL Primers: Sequence of β$_2$-microglobulin primers used in 5'–3' orientation. Sense primer B2M-5: CTC GCG CTA CTC TCT CTT TCT; Antisense primer B2M-3: TGT CGG ATT GAT GAA ACC CAG. Sequence of the AML1 and ETO-primers used in 5'–3' orientation. Sense primer: AML1-5: GAA GTG

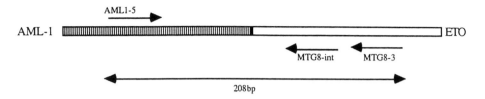

Fig. 1. Relative localization of primers used for PCR and screening.

GAA GAG GGA AAA GCT; Antisense primer MTG8-3: GGG GGA GGT GGC ATT GTT. The relative localization of primers used is shown in Fig. 1. Information about the AML1 and ETO sequences is provided (*see* Note 2).

2.4. Analysis of PCR Products

1. 2% Agarose in 1X TAE buffer: 40 mM Tris-acetate, 1 mM EDTA, 0.0001% ethidium bromide.
2. 5X Sample loading buffer: 0.25% bromophenol blue, 0.25% xylene cyanol FF, 15% Ficoll (type 400 Pharmacia) in 5X TAE.

2.5. Hybridization and Screening

1. MTG8-int primer. Sequence is shown in 5'–3' orientation (*see* Fig. 1): AGC CTA GAT TGC GTC TTC ACA TCC 10 pmol/μL.
2. 10 U/μL Polynucleotide kinase (Pharmacia).
3. 10X Kinase buffer: 500 mM Tris-HCl, pH 7.5, 100 mM MgCl$_2$ 50 mM DTT, 1 mM spermidine.
4. [γ^{32}P] ATP (3000 Ci/mmol, Amersham, Arlington Heights, IL).
5. Hybridization buffer: 0.5M sodium phosphate, pH 7.2, 7% sodium dodecylsulfate (SDS), 1 mM EDTA.
6. Sephadex G25 spin column.
7. 10 mg/mL Herringsperm DNA (Boehringer Mannheim).
8. Washing solution: 40 mM sodium phosphate, pH 7.2, 1% SDS.
9. X-Ray film (Kodak, Rochester, NY).

3. Methods

Because PCR procedure for the detection of the chimerical AML1/ETO transcript is highly sensitive, it can be used as a method for the diagnosis and detection of minimal residual disease during and after treatment *(4,7)*. Since the translocation gives rise to a chimerical AML1/ETO mRNA translation into cDNA using reverse transcriptase (RT) is necessary first. The following one step PCR is a rapid and accurate method for the detection of this chromosomal abnormality. When oligonucleotide primers derived from the AML1 and ETO cDNAs are used specific fusion transcripts can be amplified in at least 98% of

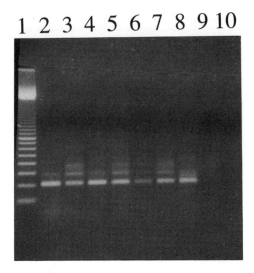

Fig. 2. Analysis of products of RT-PCR after agarose gel electrophoresis. Lane 1: 100 bp DNA molecular weight marker; Lane 2: cell line Kasumi-1; Lane 3–8: peripheral blood samples of patients with AML-M2; Lane 9: cell line Jurkat; Lane 10: dH₂O instead of RNA template.

the patients even in case of cytogenetically masked translocations. This percentage is based on a summary of data presented in recent literature *(8,14,15,16)*. Thus far only very few cases of AML-M2 carrying the t(8; 21) were reported in which the RT-PCR analysis was negative (in one out of 11 patients *[8]*; in one out of eight patients van de Locht, unpublished observation). This suggests that alternative breakpoints exist. In at least one patient, the breakpoint within AML-1 was indeed located downstream to the breakpoint cluster *(8)*. A Southern blotting procedure for the screening of genomic DNA to detect the presence of the translocation is less sensitive *(see* Note 3).

Using RT-PCR on the AML1/ETO junction in AML-M2 patient samples fragments of expected size as well as some additional slower migrating bands can be observed after agarose gel electrophoresis or on autoradiogram *(7,9,14;* and Fig. 2). This is owing to molecular diversity at the mRNA level in the AML1/ETO fusion *(17)* *(see* Note 4).

3.1. RNA Isolation

RNA is extracted using the guanidinium thiocyanate acid phenol chloroform procedure *(18)* with minor modifications.

1. Spin down 1×10^6 cells in an Eppendorf tube for 5 min at 14,000g.
2. Remove supernatant and put tubes on ice.

3. Add to the pellet: 100 μL of guanidinium thiocyanate solution containing 100 μg/mL yeast tRNA (Boehringer/Mannheim) as a carrier and vortex for 10 s, 50 μL of 2M NaAc and mix well; 500 μL of water saturated phenol and mix; and 100 μL of chloroform/isoamylalcohol (49:1), vortex well for 10 s.
4. Place tubes on ice for 10 min.
5. Centrifuge 15 min 14,000g at 4°C.
6. Transfer 400 μL of the supernatant to an Eppendorf tube containing 400 μL isopropanol and mix. Place at least 1 h at –20°C. Centrifugate 15 min 14,000g at 4°C.
7. Dissolve pellet in 150 μL GITC solution, add 150 μL isopropanol, mix and place at least 1 h at –20°C. Centrifugate for 15 min at 14,000g at 4°C and remove supernatant.
8. Wash pellet (twice) with 200 μL 75% ethanol. Centrifugate 1 min at 14,000g and remove supernatant.
9. Dry pellet 5 min in Speed-Vac.
10. Dissolve RNA in 50 μL DEPC dH$_2$O by heating 10 min at 65°C. Store RNA at –70°C.

Care must be taken to avoid RNase contamination since this will result in degradation of samples. RNA quality is assessed using a RT PCR on β$_2$-microglobulin RNA.

3.2. cDNA Synthesis

To prevent contamination, all solutions used for cDNA synthesis and the subsequent PCR are checked and aliquoted. Aerosol-resistant pipet tips are used. RNA isolations, PCR preparations, and analysis of PCR products are performed in separate parts of the laboratory. In each RT-PCR positive and negative control, RNA samples are used. Two independent RT-PCR procedures are performed on β$_2$-microglobulin and AML1/ETO, respectively.

1. In a plastic microfuge tube, mix: 8.5 μL DEPC water, 4 μL of 5X RT buffer, 0.5 μL of 25 mM dNTP, 1 μL of 100 pmol/μL random hexamers, 5 μL of RNA solution, 1 μL of 40 U/μL RNasin, and 1 μL of 200 U/μL Mo-MuLV RT.
2. Add 100 μl mineral oil to overlay the reaction.
3. Incubate for 10 min at 20°C, followed by 42°C for 45 min, and 10 min at 95°C.

Subsequently put the samples on ice and proceed to the PCR.

3.3. PCR on AML1/ETO

1. Prepare a master mix in a plastic microfuge tube. For convenience, multiply the amount of solutions used by the number of samples (n) to be analyzed exceeded by one ($n + 1$). Per sample add and mix: 55.5 μL dH$_2$O, 8 μL of 10× PCR buffer, 3 μL of AML1-5 primer, 3 μL of MTG8-3 primer, and 0.5 μL of 5 U/μL *Taq* polymerase.

2. Take 80 μL of master mix solution and add to the cDNA reaction mixture.
3. Perform PCR in a thermocycler starting with a denaturation step at 94°C for 5 min.
4. For AML1/ETO cDNA amplification this is followed by 35 cycles of: 94°C for 1.5 min, 55°C for 2 min, and 72°C for 2 min.
5. After the last cycle an additional extension phase of 10 min at 72°C is performed. Subsequently, the samples can be cooled to 4°C.

3.4. PCR on β_2-Microglobulin

1. Prepare a master mix in a plastic microfuge tube. For convenience, multiply the amount of solutions used by the number of samples (n) to be analyzed exceeded by one ($n + 1$). Per sample add and mix: 65.5 μL dH$_2$O, 8 μL of 10× PCR buffer, 3 μL of 10 pmol/μL B2M-5 primer, 3 μL of 10 pmol/μL B2M-3 primer, and 0.5 μL of 5 U/μL *Taq* polymerase.
2. Take 80 μL of master mix solution and add to the cDNA reaction mixture.
3. Perform PCR in a thermocycler starting with a denaturation step at 94°C for 5 min.
4. For β_2-microglobulin cDNA amplification the denaturation step is followed by 30 cycles of: 94°C for 30 s, 55°C for 30 s, and 72°C for 90 s.
5. In both reactions, after the last cycle an additional extension phase of 10 min at 72°C is performed. Subsequently, the samples can be cooled to 4°C.

3.5. Agarose Gel Electrophoresis and Southern Blotting

1. To each tube add: 100 μL of TE saturated chloroform and vortex briefly and spin down for a few seconds.
2. Transfer 15 μL of the upper layer to a new tube containing electrophoresis sample buffer. Mix well.
3. Load the sample onto 2% agarose gel in 1X TAE buffer containing 5 mg/mL ethidium bromide. The gel pattern can be analyzed after electrophoresis for approx 1 h at 120 V. The expected fragments are 208 bps for AML1-ETO (Fig. 2) and 130 bps for β_2-microglobulin.
4. Southern blotting can be performed according to standard procedures.

3.6. Kinasing of Oligonucleotide Primer and Hybridization of Southern Blot

An internal oligonucleotide probe MTG8-int (Fig. 1) is used to screen the Southern blot for confirmation of the AML1/ETO products (*see* Note 5).

1. In a plastic microcentrifuge tube mix: 7.0 μL dH$_2$O, 5.0 μL γ^{32}P-ATP, 5.0 μL MTG8-int primer (10 pmol/μL), 2.0 mL 10X kinase buffer, and 1.0 μL T4 polynucleotide kinase (10 U/μL).
2. Incubate at 37°C for 30 min.
3. Heat inactivate the enzyme for 5–10 min at 68°C.
4. Remove free label by G-25 spin column centrifugation.

Hybridization of the blot with the radioactively labeled primer and subsequent washing is according to standard procedures.

3.7. Interpretation of Results

Samples are regarded to be positive for AML1/ETO chimerical RNA when a hybridization signal is visible after exposure of the filters, whereas negative controls are negative and the β_2-microglobulin reaction is positive on agarose gel. Samples are regarded to be negative when no signal is visible on the auto radiogram after PCR, whereas positive controls and the β_2-microglobulin reaction are positive. This way one t(8;21) positive cell among 10^5 negative cells can be detected (*see* Note 6).

4. Notes

1. Isolation of bone marrow/blood cells: Mononuclear cells from bone marrow and peripheral blood samples are isolated by Ficoll-Hypaque centrifugation and washed with phosphate buffered saline (PBS) according to standard procedures using Percoll of a density of 1.085 g/mL.
2. AML1/ETO sequences in EMBL/Genbank: The cDNA sequences of the AML1/ETO, the AML1 and the ETO genes are present in the EMBL/Genbank. From this sequence information the primers for the PCR are derived. The accession number for the complete codons of the AML1/ETO fusion transcript is D13979 (ID number HSAMFP). The accession number for the complete codons of the human AML1 mRNA is D10570 or D90525 (ID number HSAML1). The accession numbers for the complete codons of two alternative human ETO mRNAs is D14820 (for MTG8a protein, ID number HSMTG8a) and D14821 (for MTG8b protein, ID number HSMTG8b), respectively. The two ETO mRNAs differ at approx 480 bps downstream of the ETO owing to alternative splicing *(4)*. The sequence of an AML1/ETO splicing variant was published by van de Locht et al. *(17)*.
3. Southern blot for detection of the translocation: All the breakpoints occur at random within a single intron of 25 kb between two coding exons of AML1. There is no specific localization of the breaks and the existence of a translocation hot spot seems unlikely *(3)*. A panel of probes generated from the AML1 gene and ETO gene regions flanking the breakpoint on chromosome 21 can be used to detect rearrangements in at least 85% of the patients. This percentage is based on a summary of data presented in recent literature *(3,7,8,19)*. In some patients the translocation is not detectable by cytogenetic analysis. On Southern blot these masked t(8;21) rearrangements at the AML1 locus can be detected *(16)*. The Southern blot assay allows detection of approx 5 leukemic cells per 100 normal cells.
4. Molecular diversity at the AML1/ETO fusion: An additional sequence of 68 bps was found to be present in approx 10% of the AML1/ETO cDNA molecules *(17)*. The organization of this sequence was studied at the DNA and cDNA level. It was found to be located in the ETO gene located directly upstream of the ETO exon involved in the translocation at chromosome 21. The resulting cDNA contains several stop codons downstream the AML1/ETO junction. The functional

role of this sequence, if any, is not known. Because of competition of different AML1/ETO cDNA molecules in the PCR, this variability in theory interferes with the sensitivity of the RT-PCR to detect minimal residual malignancy. As an alternative a PCR can be performed using the AML1-5 primer and a AML1/ETO breakpoint primer. This way only one AML1/ETO product is amplified. The sequence of this antisense breakpoint primer is: 5'-TGC TTC TCA GTA CGA TTT CGA-3'. For confirmation after Southern blotting an internally localized sense primer can be used. The sequence of this 821U sense primer is: 5'-AGC TTC ACT CTG ACC ATC AC-3'. The PCR conditions are the same as described in Section 3.3.

5. Nonradioactive labeling: Nonradioactive labeling of the hybridization primer is possible. Usually, a thiol-linker or aminolinker is used. Different systems are available commercially.

6. Sensitivity of the RT-PCR: Specific fusion transcripts can be detected from as little as 0.1 ng of total RNA from leukemia patients. The RT-PCR potentially allows detection of one leukemic cell among 10^4–10^5 cells without the translocation *(8)* double step PCR is even more sensitive *(4)*.

References

1. Erickson, P., Gao, J., Chang, K.-S., Look, T., Whisenant, E., Raimondi, S., Lasher, R., Trujillo, J., Rowley, J., and Drabkin, H. (1992) Identification of breakpoints in t(8;21) acute myelogenous leukemia and isolation of a fusion transcript, AML1/ETO, with similarity to Drosophila segmentation gene, runt. *Blood* **80**, 1825–1831.

2. Nisson, P. E., Watkins, P. C., and Sacchi, N. (1992) Transciptionally active chimeric gene derived from the fusion of the AML1 gene and a novel gene on chromosome 8 in t(8;21) leukemic cells. *Cancer Genet. Cytogenet.* **63**, 81–88.

3. Shimizu, K., Miyoshi, H., Kuzy, T., Nagata, J., Enomoto, K., Maseki, N., Kankeo, Y., and Ohki, M. (1992) Consistent disruption of the AML1 gene occurs within a single intron in the t(8;21) chromosomal translocation, *Cancer Res.* **52**, 6945–6948.

4. Kozu, T., Miyoshi, H., Shimizu, K., Maseki, N., Kaneko, Y., Asou, H., Kamada, N., and Ohki, M. (1993) Junctions of the AML1/MTG8(ETO) fusion are constant in t(8;21) acute myeloid leukemia detected by reverse transcription polymerase chain reaction, *Blood* **82**, 1270–1276.

5. Miyoshi, H., Shimizu, K., Kozu, T., Maseki, N., Kaneko, Y., and Ohki, M. (1991) t(8;21) breakpoints on chromosome 21 in acute myeloid leukemia are clustered within a limited region of a single gene, AML1. *Proc. Natl. Acad. Sci. USA* **88**, 10431–10434.

6. Tighe, J. E., Daga, A., and Calabi, F. (1993) Translocation breakpoints are clustered on both chromosome 8 and chromosome 21 in the t(8;21) of acute myeloid leukemia, *Blood* **81**, 592–596.

7. Nucifora, G., Birn, D. J., Erickson, P., Gao, J., LeBeau, M. M., Drabkin, H. A., and Rowley, J. D. (1993) Detection of DNA rearrangements in the AML1 and ETO loci and of an AML1/ETO fusion mRNA in patients with t(8;21) acute myeloid leukemia. *Blood* **81**, 883–888.

8. Zhang, T., Hillion, J., Tong, J.-H., Cao, Q., Chen, S.-J., Berger, R., and Chen, Z. (1994) AML1 Gene rearrangement and AML-1-ETO Gene expression as molecular markers of Acute myeloid leukemia with t(8;21), *Leukemia* **8(5),** 729–734.

9. Chang, K.-S., Fan, Y.-H., Stass, S. A., Estey, E. H., Wang, G., Trujillo, J. M., Erickson, P., and Drabkin, H. (1993) Expression of AML1-ETO fusion transcripts and detection of minimal residual disease in t(8;21)-positive acute myeloid leukemia. *Oncogene* **8,** 983–988.

10. Nucifora, G., Birn, D. J., Espinosa, R., Erickson, P., LeBeau, M., Roulston, D., McKeithan, T. W., Drabkin, H., and Rowley, J. D. (1993) Involvement of AML1 gene in the t(3;21) in therapy-related leukemia and in chronic myeloid leukemia in blast crisis. *Blood* **81,** 2728–2734.

11. Mitani, K., Ogawa, S., Tanaka, T., Miyoshi, H., Kurokawa, M., Mano, H., Yazaki, Y., Ohki, M., and Hirai, H. (1994) Generation of the AML1-EVI-1 fusion gene in the t(3;21) (q26;q22) causes blastic crisis in chronic myelocytic leukemia. *EMBO J.* **13,** 504–510.

12. Meyers, S., Downing, J. R., and Hiebert, S. W. (1993) Identification of AML-1 and the (8;21) translocation protein (AML-1/ETO) as sequence specific DNA binding proteins: the RUNT homology domain is required for DNA binding and protein–protein interaction. *Mol. Cell. Biol.* **13,** 6336–6345.

13. Asou, H., Tashiro, S., Hamamoto, K., Otsuji, A., Kita, K., and Kamada, N. (1991) Establishment of a human acute myeloid leukemia cell line (Kasumi-1) with 8;21 chromosome translocation. *Blood* **77,** 2031–2036.

14. Downing, J. R., Head, D. R., Curcio-Brint, A. M., Hulshof, M. G., Motroni, T. A., Raimondi, S. C., Carroll, A. J., Drabkin, H. A., Willman, C., Theil, K. S., Civin, C. I., and Erickson, P. (1993) An AML1/ETO Fusion transcript is consistently detected by RNA-based polymerase chain reaction in acrute myelogenous leukemia containg the (8;21) (q22;q22) translocation. *Blood* **81(11),** 2860–2865.

15. Maruyama, F., Stass, S. A., Estey, E. H., Cork, A., Masami, H., Ino, T., Freireich, E. J., Yang, P., and Chang, K.-S. (1994) Detection of AML1/ETO fusion transcript as a tool for diagnosing t(8;21) positive acute myeloid leukemia. *Leukemia* **8(1),** 40–45.

16. Maruyama, F., Yang, P., Stass, S., Cork, A., Freirich, E., Lee, M., and Chang, K. (1993) Detection of the AML1/ETO fusion transcript in the t(8;21) masked translocation in acute myelogenous leukemia. *Cancer Research* **53,** 4449–4451.

17. van de Locht, L. T. F., Smetsers, T. F. C. M., Wittebol, S., Raymakers, R. A. P., and Mensink, E. J. B. M. (1994) Molecular diversity in AML1/ETO fusion transcripts in patients with t(8;21) positive acute myeloid leukemia. *Leukemia* **8(10),** 1780–1784.

18. Puissant, C. and Houdebine, L. M. (1990) An improvement of the single-step method of RNA isolation by acid guanidium thiocyanate-phenol-chlorphorm extraction. *Biotechniques* **8,** 148–149.

19. Maseki, N., Miyoshi, H., Shimizu, K., Homma, C., Ohki, M., Sakurai, M., and Kaneko, Y. (1993) The 8;21 chromosome translocation in acute myeloid leukemia is always detectable by molecular analysis using AML1. *Blood* **81(6),** 1573–1579.

4

Analysis of the PML/RAR-α Fusion Gene in Acute Promyelocytic Leukemia by Reverse-Transcription Polymerase Chain Reaction

Technical Recommendations, Advantages, and Pitfalls

Daniela Diverio, Anna Luciano, Roberta Riccioni, Francesco Lo Coco, and Andrea Biondi

1. Introduction

Perhaps more than any other tumor marker associated with hematological neoplasia, the PML/RAR-α hybrid gene has been shown to be important in the clinical practice. This aberration is absolutely APL-specific, being found in virtually 100% of cases and in no other tumors. Secondly, it identifies a clinical entity that is unique in its response to a specific treatment, i.e., the differentiative agent all-trans retinoic acid (ATRA). As the disease frequently presents with a life-threatening hemorrhagic diathesis, its prompt recognition in order to start the specific treatment is mandatory *(1,2)*. In this respect, reverse-transcription polymerase chain reaction (RT-PCR) amplification of the specific fusion gene represents an extremely useful diagnostic tool. Finally, several groups have independently reported that RT-PCR monitoring studies of residual disease in APL provide important prognostic informations, by predicting hematologic relapse in patients who test positive during clinical remission *(3–5)*.

Based on these considerations, it appears that a standardized RT-PCR method to amplify the PML/RAR-α gene would be of considerable aid in molecular biology laboratories with prominent interest in clinical studies regarding diagnosis and monitoring of leukemia. However, in spite of its rel-

From: *Methods in Molecular Medicine, Molecular Diagnosis of Cancer*
Edited by: F. E. Cotter Humana Press Inc., Totowa, NJ

evance, the diffusion of the RT-PCR assay for PML/RAR-α in clinically oriented hematological laboratories has been relatively limited, probably owing to technical difficulties. Since 1990, we have devoted much effort to the setting up and optimization of this assay. So far it has been employed in more than 300 diagnostic and in several hundreds remission samples by functioning as referring molecular biology laboratories for the APL cases all over Italy. We report here some technical recommendations that may help to obtain reliable results when using the RT-PCR technique for diagnostic or monitoring studies in APL.

2. Solution and Materials

2.1. cDNA Synthesis

1. Random hexamers (500 μg/mL) (5' NNNNNN 3' were N = A, C, G, or T).
2. Diethylpyrocarbonate (DEPC)-treated water or bidistilled water for clinical use.
3. 5X RT buffer: 250 mM Tris-HCl, pH 8.3, 375 mM KCl, 15 mM MgCl$_2$.
4. dNTP stock: 10 mM each dATP, dGTP, dCTP, and dTTP.
5. 0.1M Dithiothreitol (DTT).
6. RNase inhibitor (40 U/μL).
7. Reverse transcriptase enzyme (200 U/μL).

2.2. PCR Mixture for FIRST PCR

1. 0.5-mL plastic tube (50-μL final vol/reaction).
2. 35 μL of water.
3. 5 μL of 10X reaction buffer: 100 mM Tris-HCl, pH 8.3, 15 mm MgCl$_2$, 500 mM KCl, 15 mM MgCl$_2$.
4. 1.85 μL of 25 mM MgCl$_2$.
5. 3.5 μL of dNTP stock (10 mM each dATP, dGTP, dCTP, and dTTP).
6. 1 μL of primer 5' (PML) 15 pmol (*see* Note 1) (M4: 5'-AGCTGCTGGAGG CTGTGGACGCGCGGTACC-3' PML exon 3 or M2: 5'-CAGTGTACGCCT TCTCCATCA-3').
7. 1 μL of primer 3' (RAR-α) 15 pmol (*see* Note 1) (R5: 5'-CCACTAGTGGTA GCCTGAGGACT-3' RAR-α exon 3).
8. 0.25 μL of Taq DNA polymerase (2.5 U/μL).
9. This makes up a volume of 48 μL and is ready for the addition of cDNA (*see* Note 2).

2.3. PCR Mixture for NESTED PCR

1. 0.5-mL plastic tube (50-μL final vol/reaction).
2. 36.75 μL water.
3. 5 μL of 10X reaction buffer: 100 mM Tris-HCl, pH 8.3, 15 mm MgCl$_2$, 500 mM KCl, 15 mM MgCl$_2$.
4. 2 μL of 1 mM MgCl$_2$.
5. 3 μL of dNTP stock (10 mM each dATP, dGTP, dCTP, and dTTP).
6. 1 μL of primer 5' (PML) M4 15 pmol.

7. 1 μL of primer 3' R8 15 pmol (R8: 5'-CAGAACTAGTGCTCTGGGTCTCAAT-3').
8. 0.25 μL of Taq DNA polymerase (2.5 U/μL).
9. This makes up a volume of 49 μL and is ready for the addition of PCR product from the FIRST PCR (*see* Note 2).

2.4. Gel Electrophoresis

1. Agarose (2% gel).
2. 10X Tris borate electrophoresis buffer (TBE): 108 g Tris-base, 55 g boric acid, and 40 mL of 0.5*M* EDTA. Make up to 1 L and autoclave. Store at room temperature.
3. Ethidium bromide (10 mg/mL stock) (*see* Note 3).

3. Methods
3.1. Collection, Preparation, and Storage of APL Samples and RNA Extraction

In contrast to most other leukemic subtypes, APL is usually a leucopenic disease at presentation. Blasts could be confined in the bone marrow (BM), and therefore the analysis of peripheral blood (PB) may be misleading, i.e., the absence of PB leukemic cells would result in false negativity. It is highly recommended to preferentially analyze BM specimens either at diagnosis or during the follow-up, with the only exception of the rare microgranular (variant form)—M3v—which is frequently hyperleukocytic *(1,2)*. Given not only to the low number of blasts, but particularly to the frequent rapid clotting of the diagnostic samples, the availability of good quality RNA may be difficult. Clotting leads to the release of lysosomal enzymes, which may cause damage to RNA integrity *(5,6)*. Samples should therefore be processed as soon as possible by isolating the mononuclear fraction (through a Ficoll-Hypaque gradient centrifugation) from the other blood components. If RNA is not immediately extracted, cells can be resuspended in a solution of 4*M* guanidium thiocyanate to prevent the action of nucleases and then stored for unlimited periods of time at –20 or –70°C. By using these precautions and working with RNAase free solutions and disposable materials, we have been able to obtain good quality RNA in at least 95% of cases. When samples are to be sent from other institutions to reference laboratories, we suggest to locally follow the detailed rules for specimens collection and storage, and to ship the vials containing the frozen mononuclear cells resuspended in GTC. Although good quality RNA to analyze other disease-specific genetic lesions may be obtained from stored whole blood, the isolation and storage in GTC of promyelocytic blasts is, at least in our experience, more effective in protecting the RNA integrity. (Alternatively, several laboratories used to store a dry pellet of isolated mononuclear cells with no GTC solution, but this procedure may lead to more frequent RNA degradation in the specific case of APL.) Both most commonly used RNA extraction techniques, i.e., the Chomczynsky and Sacchi guanidium thiocyanate *(7)* and the Cesium Chloride (CsC1) methods *(8)* are equally effective to obtain sufficient RNA for the analysis. However, the former is recommended when a rapid extraction is needed while cleaner (more DNA-free) RNA is obtained using ultracentrifugation on a CsC1 gradient. The yield of RNA and its degree of protein contamination is determined by spectrophotometry. Finally, we suggest to always assess the RNA quality by running an aliquot on a formaldehyde gel.

3.2. cDNA Synthesis

The generation of the PML-RAR-α cDNA by reverse transcription is carried out according to established procedures using commercially available enzymes and reagents *(8)* and is also presented more fully in other chapters. In our hands, the efficiency of the various enzymes shows only slight differences with comparable cDNA yields. As primers, we use random hexamers, but RAR-α complementary 3' oligos or dT tails are equally effective.

1. In a 0.5-mL microtube mix: 1 μL random hexamer as primers and 5 μL DEPC-treated water.
2. Add 2 μL RNA 0.5 μg/μL.
3. Incubate at 70°C for 10 min.
4. Add 4 μL of 5X RT buffer.
5. Add 4 μL of mixed dNTP stock.
6. Add 2 μL of 0.1M DTT.
7. Add 1 μL of RNase inhibitor.
8. Finally add 1 μL of RT (200 U/μL) at room temperature.
9. Mix the reagents very well.
10. Incubate at 37°C for 60 min, at 99°C for 5 min, and at 5°C for 5 min.
11. An aliquot of 2 μL of cDNA is then diluted with 48 μL of FIRST PCR mixture (*see* Section 2.2.).

3.3. FIRST PCR

1. After an initial denaturation at 95°C for 2 min, incubate at: 95°C for 20 s (denaturation), 50°C for 20 s (annealing), and 72°C for 20 s (extension).
2. Repeat this cycle for a total of 30 on an automated heat block (DNA thermal cycler).
3. At the end, 1 μL of FIRST PCR product is used for a second round of amplification.

3.4. Nested (Second Round) PCR

A half nested approach is used by employing in the second PCR round an internal RAR-α exon 3 oligo (R8), and the same 5' primer (M4 or M2) as in the first step. Such a procedure is required at diagnosis or whenever the PML breakpoint type is still to be determined. Given to alternative splicing on PML, more than one band is visualized on the ethidium bromide gel in case of *bcr*

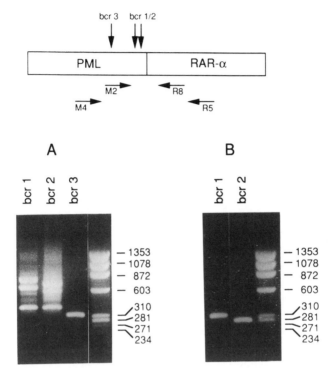

Fig. 1. PCR amplification of the PML/RAR--α in APL: identification of "universal" primers.

types 1 or 2 (located in intron 6 and exon 6, respectively, also referred to as "long transcript"), as shown in Fig. 1. Alternatively, in cases with *bcr* type 3 (located in intron 3, "short transcript"), a single band is amplified using these primers. When the occurrence of *bcr* 1–2 is suggested by the amplification of several bands and a *bcr*3 has been ruled out, a downstream primer closer to the breakpoint (located on PML exon 5) is used to amplify a single fragment (Fig. 1B). Once the *bcr* type has been identified for each case, PCR follow-up experiments may be carried out with the appropriate primers always allowing the visualization of a single band.

1. Add 1 µL of FIRST PCR product to 49 µL of second round of amplification mixture.
2. Heat the samples and run 30 cycles on an automated heat block as done for the FIRST PCR at the same cycling temperatures.

3.5. Gel Electrophoresis

1. A 2% gel is made by boiling 2 g agarose/10 mL of TBE (1X).
2. Cool to approx 50°C and add 10 µL of ethidium bromide/100 mL.

3. Pour the agarose into an appropriate casting tray. (Minigels are usually adequate with a slim 1-mm comb.)
5. After setting, add 1X TBE solution to the gel tank.
4. At the end of PCR reaction, take 10-μL of PCR mixture and run on the 2% agarose gel stained. The amplification product will bind with the ethidium bromide and can then be readily visualized under a UV lamp (*see* Notes 4–6).

4. Notes

1. The location of PML and RAR-α oligoprimers and PCR conditions are described in detail in several published manuscripts *(6, 9–13)*. The use of 5' primers on PML exon 3 (M4) or exon 5 (M2) and 3' RAR-α exon 3 (R5) is the most commonly used first-step strategy.
2. Always store the prepared PCR reaction mixture on ice prior to adding the appropriate cDNA. It is advisable to make up the reaction mixture in batches and then aliquot the 48-μL into individual tubes for PCR.
3. Ethidium bromide should always be handled with extreme care, wearing gloves as it readily binds DNA and as such is carcinogenic. It should not be added to very hot agarose, as this will create toxic ethidium bromide vapors (add at an approximate temperature of 50°C).
4. The PCR product should be run alongside a DNA size marker. Useful size markers include ΦX1 ladder, 123-bp ladder, 100-bp ladder, and 1-kb ladder, all of which are commercially available from Gibco-BRL (Gaithersburg, MD). A brophenol blue loading buffer is usually used.
5. Positive and negative controls are to be used in each experiment in order to verify the efficiency of the reaction and to rule out possible contaminations. As a positive control, the APL derived NB4 cell line is frequently used. Alternatively, an APL diagnostic RNA with known PML/RAR-α fusion product may be included in the experiment. Similarly to any other negative control test, this is done by mixing all the reagents without the sample ("water lane"). As we have discussed, the integrity of the RNA is one of the most crucial issues in the RT-PCR analysis of APL. In addition to the visualization of the extracted RNA on the formaldehyde gel, the amplification of a cDNA fragment is required in order to (1) confirm RNA integrity and (2) evaluate the efficiency of the reverse transcription step. Such reaction, to be always performed in all experiments, requires careful attention in the choice of the gene to be amplified as well as in the location of primers. Indeed, this is one of the most discussed issues in all PCR experiments. Also, there is considerable variability of the genes selected for this purpose in different laboratories. As a general rule, it would be reasonable to avoid using housekeeping or constitutively expressed genes and choose preferentially one of the two genes involved in the translocation. Secondly, the location primers should always encompass the breakpoint in order that single copy of template gene per chromosome would be present at diagnosis either for the control or for the translocated allele *(14)*. In other words, this would allow a theoretically identical copy number of templates for each reaction (PML/RAR-α vs normal allele)

in a case with 100% leukemic cells. However, variations in the RNA stability or other factors influencing the transcription rates may also influence the amount of normal vs translocated allele copies. We used to amplify an RAR-α fragment, including exons 2–3, with the (R2: 5'-GCTCTGACCACTCTCCAGCA-3') primer located upstream with respect to RAR-α breakpoint and a primer located downstream of it (R5: 5'-CCACTAGTGGTAGCCTGAGGACT-3' or R8: 5'-CAG AACTAGTGCTCTGGGTCTCAAT-3').

6. To determine the sensitivity of the reaction, dilution experiments have been performed by mixing NB4 RNA (or RNA from APL) with a non-APL leukemic cell line, as reported *(10)*. In our hands, the detection level of MRD using this technique is around 10^{-4} and is similar to that found by others. As compared to other RT-PCR used to detect leukemia-associated hybrid genes (such as the BCR/ABL), such sensitivity seems to be lower. These differences are probably owing to a number of factors, including lower expression and greater instability of the PML/RAR-α hybrid with respect to other fusion genes.

7. For the future, in even for the most experienced molecular biology laboratory, the setting of a PCR test to amplify a novel translocation requires a variable number of attempts in order to find out the best experimental conditions. In the specific case of APL, we have seen that even before the setting of the reaction, a number of precautions are needed to obtain good quality RNA. Again we would emphasize that an RNA yield is probably the main problem when dealing with APL.

Several aspects should be examined in more detail in the near future to improve the technique. These may include the use of other RNA protective agents, the setting of more efficient reverse transcription, the design of other oligonucleotides allowing a higher sensitivity of the assay, and the use of signal enhancers. The improvement of sensitivity levels is perhaps the most important goal for the near future. In fact, although most PCR negative patients evaluated in remission with the currently available methods are likely to become long-term survivors, others have been reported to convert to PCR positive and relapse. Therefore, it appears that a more efficient RT-PCR assay in remission could identify more patients at risk of relapse who may benefit of additional therapy.

References

1. Warrel, R. P., Jr., de Thé, H., Wang, Z.-Y., and Degos, L. (1993) Acute promyelocytic leukemia. *N. Engl. J. Med.* **329**, 177–89.
2. Grignani, F., Fagioli, M., Alcalay, M., Longo, L., Pandolfi, P. P., Donti, E., Biondi, A., Lo Coco, F., Grignani, F., and Pelicci, P. G. (1994) Acute promyelocytic leukemia: from genetics to treatment. *Blood* **83**, 10–25.
3. Lo Coco, F., Diverio, D., Pandolfi, P. P., Biondi, A., Rossi, V., Avvisati, G., Rambaldi, A., Arcese, W., Petti, M. C., Meloni, G., Mandelli, F., Grignani, F., Masera, G., Barbui, T., and Pelicci, P. G. (1992) Molecular evaluation of residual disease as predictor of relapse in acute promyelocytic leukemia. *Lancet* **340**, 1437,1438.
4. Chang, K. S., Lu, J., Wang, G., Trujillo, J. M., Estey, E., Cork, A., Chu, D. T., Freireich, E. J., and Stass, S. A. (1992) The t(15; 17) breakpoint in acute

promyelocytic leukemia cluster within two different sites of the myl gene. Targets for the detection of minimal residual disease by polymerase chain reaction. *Blood* **79**, 554.

5. Miller, W. H., Jr., Levine, K., DeBlasio, A., Frankel, S. R., Dmitrovsky, E., and Warrel, R. P., Jr. (1993) Detection of minimal residual disease in acute promyelocytic leukemia by reverse transcription polymerase chain reaction assay for the PML/RAR-α fusion mRNA. *Blood* **82**, 1689–1694.

6. Miller, W. H., Jr., Kakizuka, A., Frankel, S. R., Warrel, R. P., Jr., De Blasio, A., Levine, K., Evans, R. M., and Dimitrovsky, E. (1992) Reverse transcription polymerase chain reaction for the rearranged retinoic acid receptor alpha clarifies diagnosis and detects minimal residual disease in acute promyelocytic leukemia. *Proc. Natl. Acad. Sci. USA* **89**, 2694.

7. Chomczynsky, P. and Sacchi, N. (1987) Single step method of RNA isolation by guanidium thiocyanate-phenol-chloroform extraction. *Anal. Biochem.* **162**, 156–158.

8. Maniatis, T., Fritsch, E. F., and Sambrook, J. (1982) *Molecular Cloning: A Laboratory Manual.* Cold Spring Harbor Laboratory, Cold Spring Harbor, NY.

9. Pandolfi, P. P., Alcalay, M., Fagioli, M., Zangrilli, D., Mencarelli, A., Diverio, D., Biondi, A., Lo Coco, F., Rambaldi, A., Grignani, F., Rochette-Egly, C., Gaube, M. P., Chambon, P., and Pelicci, P. G. (1992) Genomic variability and alternative splicing generate multiple PML/RAR-α transcripts that encode aberrant PML proteins and PML/RAR-α isoforms in acute promyelocytic leukaemia. *EMBO J.* **1**, 1397.

10. Biondi, A., Rambaldi, A., Pandolfi, P. P., Rossi, V., Giudici, G., Alcalay, M., Lo Coco, F., Diverio, D., Pogliani, E. M., Lanzi, E. M., Mandelli, F., Masera, G., Barbui, T., and Pelicci, P. G. (1992) Molecular monitoring of the myl/RAR-α fusion gene in acute preomyelocytic leukemia by polymerase chain reaction. *Blood* **80**, 492.

11. Castaigne, S., Balitrand, N., de Thé, H., Dejean, A., Degos, L., and Chomienne, C. (1992) A PML-Retinoic acid receptor alpha fusion transcripts is constantly detected by RNA-based polymerase chain reaction in acute promyelocytic leukemia. *Blood* **79**, 3110.

12. Chen, S.-J., Chen, Z., Chen, A., Tong, J.-H., Dong, S., Wang, Z.-Y., Waxman, S., and Zelent, A. (1992) Occurrence of distinct PML-RAR-α isoforms in patients with acute promyelocytic leukemia detected by reverse transcriptase/polymerase chain reaction. *Oncogene* **7**, 1223.

13. Huang, W., Sun, G.-L., Li, X.-S., Cao, Q., Lu, Y., Jang, G.-S., Zhang, F.-Q., Chai, J.-R., Wang, Z.-Y., Waxman, S., Chen, Z., and Chen, S.-J. (1993) Acute promyelocytic leukemia: relevance of two major PML-RAR-α isoforms and detection of minimal residual disease by reverse transcriptase-polymerase chain reaction to predict relapse. *Blood* **82**, 1264–1269.

14. Melo, J. V., Kent, N. S., Yan, X. -H., and Goldman, J. M. (1994) Controls for reverse transcriptase-polymerase chain reaction amplification of BCR-ABL transcripts. *Blood* **84**, 3984–3986.

5

RT-PCR Analysis of Breakpoints Involving the MLL Gene Located at 11q23 in Acute Leukemia

Chris F. E. Pocock and Finbarr E. Cotter

1. Introduction

Chromosome rearrangements of chromosome 11 at band 11q23 are detected in a high proportion of infant leukemias (<1 yr) as well as childhood and adult acute leukemias of both myeloid and lymphoid types. Molecular and cytogenetic analysis of these tumors has shown that 7–10% of acute lymphoblastic, and 5–6% of acute nonlymphocytic leukemias are involved in this way (1). Leukemias with rearrangements of band 11q23 typically are CD10⁻, exhibit biphenotypic or mixed-lineage phenotype, and have a poor response to chemotherapy (2). The gene on chromosome 11 involved in the 11q23 rearrangement has been cloned recently (3,4) and characterized. It is known as MLL (or ALL-1, HRX, HTRX), the gene encodes a 3969-amino acid polypeptide showing areas of homology to the *Drosophila trithorax* gene, a putative regulator of homeotic genes in segment determination (5). The MLL gene is large and complex, containing two DNA-binding domains consisting of three AT-hook motifs and two multiple zinc-finger domains, and thus has the characteristics of a transcription factor likely to be involved in the regulation of gene expression.

The MLL gene has been described as "promiscuous" because of the large number of reciprocal partners involved in the translocation. Other chromosomes that have been implicated include 4, 9, 19, 1, 2, 5, 6, 10, 14, 15, 17, 22, and X. Correspondingly a panel of primers required for screening of the translocations must be large to encompass the increasing number of possible reciprocal partners. The majority of translocations, however, involve chromosomes

From: *Methods in Molecular Medicine, Molecular Diagnosis of Cancer*
Edited by: F. E. Cotter Humana Press Inc., Totowa, NJ

4, 9, and 19 and methods are described in Chapter 5 enabling the detection of these abnormalities by a RNA-based PCR method.

The use of RNA, rather than genomic DNA, in PCR assays is required. The method relies on the ability of the enzyme reverse transcriptase (a retroviral enzyme not normally found in mammalian cells) to generate double-stranded DNA from a mRNA template. This complementary cDNA represents the transcribed regions of the gene with the introns spliced out. The use of random hexamers as primers (*see* Section 2.2. later) enables a representative copy of the entire transcribed sequences in the genome to be analyzed in the form of cDNA. Alternatively, if a single area of the cDNA is to be investigated then a single specific primer positioned just 5' upstream from the area of interest can be used to generate multiple copies only of the cDNA area of interest. The disadvantage is that if further sequences elsewhere need to be examined, for example a control, noninvolved sequence, then the use of a specific primer means there is no representation of these other sequences in the cDNA copy.

Rearrangements of the MLL gene have breakpoints clustering within the regions containing exons 5–9 *(6,7)* (Fig. 1). However, many of these exons are separated by large introns often containing regions of Alu repeats. For example, the intron between exons 8 and 9 (a region of high frequency of breakpoints) spans 3.7 kb *(8)*, and thus is inaccessible to conventional PCR methodology. If an RNA based technique is used then repetitive intron sequences are spliced out during the production of mRNA and the target area for PCR amplification can be reduced approx 10-fold. The cDNA sequence for MLL exons 5–9 spans only ~650 bp, easily accessible to conventional PCR methods. The location of breakpoints in the reciprocal partners allows identification of rearranged sequences utilizing amplification of less than 800 bp in the majority of cases.

Historically, rearrangements at chromosome band 11q23 have been investigated using the techniques of conventional cytogenetics and Southern blotting. Both these techniques are time-consuming and labor intensive. Adequate metaphases for karyotyping by G-banding are often difficult to obtain in infant leukemic samples, and the sensitivity of chromosome analysis and Southern blotting is probably only in the order of 1 in 100 cells. Although the use of fluorescence *in situ* hybridization (FISH) undoubtedly has increased the sensitivity of chromosome analysis, allowing the examination of interphase as well as metaphase cells, it remains demanding in terms of time and effort. The use of modern techniques for the rapid extraction of mRNA from small samples and the use of an RT-based PCR technique based on a panel of different primers theoretically allows the detection or otherwise of rearrangements of the MLL gene within 24 h. Furthermore, the sensitivity of the technique is probably in the range of 1 in 100,000 cells, thus allowing it potentially to be used as a screen for minimal residual disease.

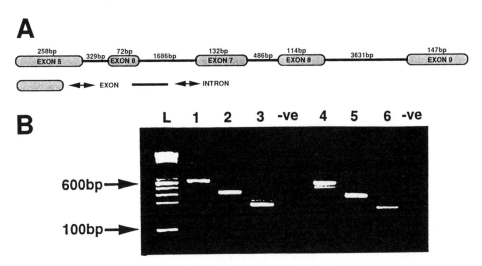

Fig. 1. (A) Graphic representation of MLL breakpoint cluster region. The total region is –7 kb in size of which –700 bp is exon sequence. **(B)** 2% Agarose gel of amplification products across MLL/AF-4 breakpoint in two patients with t(4;11). Patient A: lane 1, MLL exon 5 – AF-4 (615 bp); lane 2, MLL exon 6 – AF-4 (415 bp); lane 3, MLL exon 7 – AF-4 (325 bp). (BP. MLL exon 8/9; AF-4 Position C). Patient B: lane 4, MLL exon 5 – AF-4 (580 bp); lane 5, MLL-exon 6 – AF-4 (380 bp); lane 6, MLL exon 7 – AF-4 (290 bp). (BP MLL exon 7/8; AF-4 Position B). Figures in parentheses are predicted band sizes from cDNA data; L = 100 bp ladder (Gibco Brl), –ve = controls.

2. Materials

2.1. RNA Isolation

All solutions and glassware should be DEPC treated to remove RNases.

1. Guanidinium-isothiocyanate solution (GITC): $4M$ guanidinium-isothiocyanate, 25 mM sodium citrate pH 7.0, 0.5% N-lauroyl sarcosine, and 0.1M β-mercaptoethanol.
2. 10 mg/mL Yeast t-RNA (Boehringer/Mannheim, Mannheim Germany).
3. $2M$ Sodium acetate, pH 4.0.
4. Water-saturated phenol.
5. Chloroform.
6. Isoamylalcohol.
7. Isopopanol.
8. DEPC-treated dH$_2$O.

2.2. cDNA Synthesis

1. 200 U/µL Mo-MLV reverse transcriptase (Gibco/BRL, Gaithersburg, MD).
2. 5X Reverse transcriptase buffer: 250 mM Tris-HCl, pH 8.3, 375 mM KCl, 15 mM MgCl$_2$.

Table 1
Primer Sequences[a]

Primer	Sequence, 5'–3'	Length, bp
Exon 5 sense	CCTGAATCCAAAC AGGCCACCACT	24
Exon 6 sense	CGCCAACTATCCC TGTAAAAC	22
Exon 7 sense	AACCACCTCCGGTC AATAAGCA	22
Exon 9 antisense	GATGTTGCCTTCCA CAAACGTGAC	24
AF-4 antisense	TCACTGAGCTGAA GGTCGTCTTC	23
AF-9 antisense	CTTGTCACATTCAC CATTCTT	21
ENL antisense 1	TCCACGAAGTGCT GGATGTCACAT	24
ENL antisense 2	CTCGGGGCCGCGG ACAAACACCAT	24
AF-X antisense	GCTGCCTGACCACT TGGCAAAGT	23

[a]Oligonucleotide sequences for amplification of fusion cDNAs involved in t(4;11)-AF-4, t(11;19)-ENL, 5(9;11)-AF-9 and t(X;11)-AF-X. Includes primers for amplification of exons 5 and 6 to exon 9 as controls. (S = sense; AS = antisense).

3. 100 mM DTT.
4. dNTP mixture of 25 mM of each nucleotide (Pharmacia, Uppsala, Sweden).
5. 100 pmol/μL Random hexamers (5' NNNNN 3') (Pharmacia).
6. 40 U/μL RNasin RNase inhibitor (Promega, Madison, WI).

2.3. PCR

1. 10X PCR buffer: 500 mM KCl, 100 mM Tris-HCl, pH 8.3, 1.0% v/v Triton X-100, 1.5 mM MgCl$_2$.
2. 5 U/μL *Taq* Polymerase.
3. 10 pmol/μL Primers: sequence of primers used in 5' to 3' orientation are shown in Table 1.

2.4. Analysis of PCR Products

1. 2% Agarose in 1X TAE buffer (40 mM Tris-acetate, 1 mM EDTA, 0.0001% ethidium bromide).
2. 5X Sample loading buffer: 0.25% bromophenol blue, 0.25% xylene cyanol FF, 15% Ficoll (type 400 Pharmacia) in 5X TAE.

3. Methods

3.1. Isolation of mRNA

Often it is desirable to have a method based on small volumes (as little as 25 μL) of whole blood. Many of the commercially available kits for mRNA or polyA RNA have such as facility, and provide a rapid method for extraction of adequate amounts of mRNA for RT-PCR. However, because of the gross hyperleucocytosis often seen in these leukemias, Ficoll-gradient isolation of leukemic blasts can be performed followed by aliquoting to allow for future experimentation as well as mRNA production. An aliquot of 1×10^6 cells extracted from blood is usually adequate for a panel of RT-PCR experiments. RNA is extracted as previously described (Chapter 3 by Mensink) and as indicated in the following.

1. Spin down 1×10^6 cells in an Eppendorf tube for 5 min at 3030g.
2. Remove supernatant and put tubes on ice.
3. Add to the pellet: 100 μL of guanidinium thiocyanate solution containing 100 μg/μL yeast tRNA (Boehringer/Mannheim) as a carrier and vortex for 10 sec, 50 μL of 2M NaAc and mix well; 500 μL of water saturated phenol and mix; and 100 μL of chloroform/isoamylalcohol (49:1), and vortex well for 10 s.
4. Place tubes on ice for 10 min.
5. Centrifuge 15 min 14,000g at 4°C.
6. Transfer 400 μL of the supernatant to an Eppendorf tube containing 400 μL isopropanol and mix. Place at least 1 h at –20°C. Centrifugate 15 min 14,000g at 4°C.
7. Dissolve pellet in 150 μL GITC solution, add 150 μL isopropanol, mix, and place at least 1 h at –20°C. Centrifugate for 15 min at 14,000g at 4°C and remove supernatant.
8. Wash pellet (twice) with 200 μL 75% ethanol. Centrifuge 1 min at 14,000g and remove supernatant.
9. Dry pellet 5 min in Speed-Vac.
10. Dissolve RNA in 50 μL DEPC dH$_2$O by heating 10 min at 65°C. Store RNA at –70°C.

3.2. Preparation of Complementary DNA (cDNA)

1. Primer annealing. Add the following to a 0.5-mL Eppendorf tube: 1 μL random hexamer, 3 μL mRNA (100 ng–5 μg), and 7 μL sterile distilled water. Place in a thermal cycler and heat to 70°C for 10 min followed by a quick chill on ice.
2. cDNA generation. Then add to the preceding mixture: 4 μL of reverse transcription 5X buffer, 1 μL dNTPs (10 mmol dATP, 10 mmol dCTP, 10 mmol dGTP, 10 mmol dTTP), 1 μL 0.1M DTT, and 1 μL RNasin. Equilibrate at room temperature for 2 min, then place in a thermal cycler at 37°C for 1 h. Heat to 95°C for 10 min then place on ice. Use 1–2 μL/50 μL PCR reaction, or store at –20°C for future use. Different versions of reverse transcriptase are available from other manufacturers, generally utilizing similar reaction protocols to those described here.

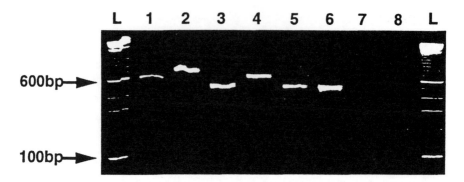

Fig. 2. 2% Agarose gel showing heterogeneity among eight patients with a t(4;11) regarding sizes of fusion amplification product using MLL exon 5 sense and AF-4 antisense primers. Lanes 1 and 4, (620 bp)-MLL exon 7/8: AF-4 position A; lane 2, (690 bp)-MLL exon 8/9: AF-4 position B; lanes 3, 5, 6, and 8, (500 bp) MLL exon 7/8: AF-4 position A; lane 7, (490 bp)-MLL exon 6/7: AF-4 position A. Figures in parentheses are predicted band sizes from cDNA data. L = 100 bp ladder (Gibco, Brl).

3.3. Amplification of cDNA

Using a 500 μL plastic tube, place 2 μL of the cDNA generated into 5 μL of 10X PCR reaction buffer together with 1 U of *Taq* polymerase enzyme, 2.5 μL of each of the oligonucleotide pairs (*see* Table 1) and 1 μL of each dNTPs, making the final volume up to 50 μL with sterile water. Mineral oil is layered over the reaction mixture and the tubes placed into the thermal cycler. The cycling program consists of 94°C for 5 min; 55°C for 45 s (72°C for 1 min; 94°C for 30 s; and 55°C for 45 s for a total of 30 cycles). Final extension is at 72°C for 10 min. (Fig. 2).

3.4. Analysis of PCR Products

1. Four microliters of PCR product is mixed with 1 μL of 5X loading buffer.
2. Load the PCR product and buffer into a well of the 2% agarose gel in TAE. Load an appropriate DNA marker (100 bp, 123 bp, or ΦXI DNA markers, Gibco-BRL) alongside.
3. Electropherese for approx 1 h at a voltage in the region of 100 V.
4. Visualize by placing the gel on a UV light box. Chimeric fusion mRNAs across the cDNA breakpoint junction may be determined by the presence or absence of a PCR band of the appropriate size on the agarose gel (*see* Notes 1–3). These are listed in Table 2. The breakpoints cluster in the region of exons 5–9 on chromosome 11 (*see* Further Reading at end of chapter).

Table 2
Expected Sizes of Amplification Products[a]

Antisense primer	Exon 5 sense	Exon 6 sense
AF-4, exon 6/7 break		
Breakpoint A	490	290
Breakpoint b	450	250
Breakpoint C	340	240
AF-4, exon 7/8 break		
Breakpoint A	620	420
Breakpoint B	580	380
Breakpoint C	500	300
AF-4, exon 8/9 break		
Breakpoint A	740	540
Breakpoint B	690	490
Breakpoint C	615	415
AF-9		
Exon 6/7 break	310	110
Exon 7/8 break	440	240
Exon 8/9 break	560	360
ENL		
Exon 6/7 break	350	150
Exon 7/8 break	480	280
Exon 8/9 break	590	390
AF-X		
Exon 6/7 break	510	310
Exon 7/8 break	640	440
Exon 8/9 break	755	555

[a]Predicted sizes of amplification products from MLL exons 5 and 6 (sense), to exon 9 (antisense, cDNA control) and the AF-4, AF-9, ENL, and AF-X genes (antisense). Comparison with band sizes on agarose gels can pinpoint breakpoints in individual patients. (Sizes given are to the nearest 10 bp.) MLL breakpoint locations 6/7, 7/8, and 8/9 are the most frequent.

4. Notes

1. Amplification products involving the t(4;11) may produce two or more bands owing to alternative splicing of the AF-4 gene.
2. Amplifications should be accompanied with appropriate positive control to ensure integrity of cDNA (e.g., amplification of exon 5 sense with exon 9 antisense).
3. Primers for different exons of MLL do not necessarily start at the beginning of each exon. Therefore, amplification sizes differ from those predicted purely from exon size.

References

1. Raimondi, S. (1993) Current status of cytogenetic research in childhood acute lymphoblastic leukemia. *Blood* **81,** 2237–2251.
2. Chen, C.-S., Sorensen, P., Domer, P., Reaman, G., Korsmeyer, S., Heerema, N., Hammond, G., and Kersey, J. (1993) Molecular rearrangements on chromosome 11q23 predominate in infant acute lymphoblastic leukemia and are associated with specific biological variables and poor outcome. *Blood* **81,** 2386–2393.
3. Djabali, M., Selleri, L., Parry, P., Bower, M., Young, B., and Evans, G. (1992) A trithorax-like gene is interrupted by chromosome 11q23 translocations in acute leukaemias. *Nature Genet.* **2,** 113–118.
4. McCabe, N., Burnett, R., Gill, H., Thirman, M., Mbangkollo, D., Kipiniak, M., van Melle, E., Ziemin-van der Poel, S., Rowley, J., and Diaz, M. (1992) Cloning of cDNAs of the MLL gene that detect DNA rearrangements and altered RNA transcripts in human leukemic cells with 11q23 translocations. *Proc. Natl. Acad. Sci. USA* **89,** 11,794–11,798.
5. Mazo, A., Huang, D.-H., Mozer, B., and Dawid, I. (1990) The trithorax gene, a trans-acting regulator of the bithorax complex in Drosophila, encodes a protein with zinc-binding domains. *Proc. Natl. Acad. Sci. USA* **87,** 2112–2116.
6. Corral, J., Forster, A., Thompson, S., Lambert, F., Kaneko, Y., Slater, R., Kories, W.-G., van der Schoot, C., Ludwig, W.-D., Karpas, A., Pocock, C., Cotter, F., and Rabbitts, T. (1993) Acute leukemias of different lineages have similar MLL gene fusions encoding related chimeric proteins resulting from chromosomal translocation. *Proc. Natl. Acad. Sci. USA* **90,** 8538–8542.
7. Yamamoto, K., Seto, M., Iida, S., Komatsu, H., Kamada, N., Kojima, S., Kodera, Y., Nakazawa, S., Saito, H., Takahashi, T., and Ueda, R. (1994) A reverse transcriptase-polymerase chain reaction detects heterogeneous chimeric mRNAs in leukemias with 11q23 abnormalities. *Blood* **83,** 2912–2921.
8. Gu, Y., Alder, H., Nakamura, T., Schichman, S., Prasad, R., Canaani, O., Saito, H., Croce, C., and Canaani, E. (1994) Sequence analysis of the breakpoint cluster region in the All-1 gene involved in acute leukemia. *Cancer Res.* **54,** 2327–2330.

Further Reading

Blumberg, D. (1987). Creating a ribonuclease-free environment, in *Methods in Enzymology* (Berger, S. and Kimmel, A., eds.), Academic, London.

Maniatis, T., Fritsch, E. F., and Sambrook, J. (1982) *Molecular Cloning: A Laboratory Manual.* Cold Spring Harbor Laboratory Press, Cold Spring Harbor, NY, pp. 387–389.

Krug, M. and Berger, S. (eds.) (1987). First strand cDNA synthesis primed with oligo dT, in *Methods in Enzymology* (Berger, S. and Kimmel, A., eds.), Academic, London.

6

Polymerase Chain Reaction for Detection of the t(14;18) Translocation in Lymphomas

Peter W. M. Johnson

1. Introduction

The t(14;18) (q21;q32) translocation was originally identified as occurring in follicular low-grade non-Hodgkin's lymphomas of B-cell origin in 1978 *(1)*, and has been found in up to 85% of cases subsequently *(2–4)*. The translocation appears to arise at the pre-B-cell stage in the bone marrow when VDJ recombination usually occurs *(5)*, so that the *Bcl*-2 gene on chromosome 18 is connected to the 5' end of one of the six J_H segments of the immunoglobulin heavy chain locus on chromosome 14 *(6)*. The result of this is the constitutional upregulation of *Bcl*-2 expression *(7,8)*, which results in the suppression of apoptotic cell death among the population carrying the abnormality *(9)*. It is suggested that this disrupts the normal process by which B-cell clones are eliminated during affinity maturation in germinal centers *(10)*, thereby giving rise to an expanded B-lymphocyte pool in which further lymphomagenic events can supervene.

The *Bcl*-2 gene has a structure of 3 exons with large introns covering a span of at least 230 kilobases *(11)*. The great majority of translocations involve breakpoints within two cluster regions—the major breakpoint region (MBR) *(6)* lying within the 3' untranslated region of the third exon and the minor cluster region (MCR) in an intronic segment at least 20 kb 3' to this *(12)*. Both these translocations leave the open reading frame intact so that the *Bcl*-2 gene product is thought to be of normal structure, although there is one report of mutations detected in cases of lymphoma bearing the t(14;18) *(13)*.

The t(14;18) is shown schematically in Fig. 1, with a translocation involving the MBR region in *Bcl*-2 and the Jh4 segment in the immunoglobulin locus illustrated.

From: *Methods in Molecular Medicine, Molecular Diagnosis of Cancer*
Edited by: F. E. Cotter Humana Press Inc., Totowa, NJ

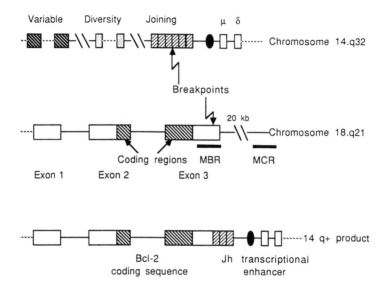

Fig. 1. Representation of the t(14;18).

The clustering of the breakpoints involved in the t(14;18) make this rear-rangement particularly suitable for detection by PCR in genomic DNA. Prim-ers have been designed to hybridize to segments on either side of the translocation in both the 14q+ and 18q– derivatives: For the 14q+ primers to the 5' section of the MBR or MCR region are used with a primer to the repeti-tive consensus sequence that lies 3' to each of the six joining segment exons (Fig. 2) *(14–16)*. For the 18q– primers to the 3' section of the MBR or MCR are used with a primer containing a heptamer from the sequence flanking unrearranged diversity segments *(17)*.

Although PCR amplification will not detect the few breakpoints lying out-side the cluster regions it offers several advantages over the alternative meth-ods of detection such as Southern blotting, pulsed-field gel electrophoresis, or classical cytogenetics. In particular, the sensitivity of PCR allows the detection of very low copy numbers of the translocation, and it permits direct sequence analysis to be carried out upon the reaction products. This latter is especially helpful in eliminating false-positive results since the variety of breakpoints within the clusters, together with the variable insertion of "N" regions or even fragments of diversity region chromatin *(17)* result in a considerable range of size of amplified PCR products. Individual t(14;18) clones may be distin-guished to some extent by speed of migration on agarose gels but more specific still is the analysis of the sequence of nucleotides up to and across the breakpoints, which is rarely, if ever, the same in two clones *(17–19)*.

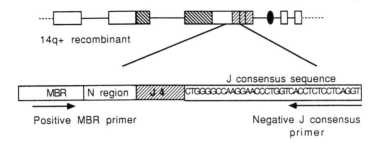

Fig. 2. PCR amplification of the 14q+ MBR breakpoint.

Some doubts have been raised regarding the use of the t(14;18) as a marker of residual lymphoma. The translocation, as well as being found at lower frequencies in other lymphoid tumors such as large cell lymphoma, immunoblastic lymphoma *(20)* and Hodgkin's disease *(21,22)*, can also be detected by PCR in benign hyperplastic tonsils *(23,24)* and the peripheral circulating B-cells of normal blood donors *(25)*. It has been shown in addition that patients with prolonged remissions following treatment of follicular lymphoma may have a persistently demonstrable presence of the original t(14;18) clone without developing recurrent disease *(26–28)*. These findings give particular importance to the use of sequencing from the PCR. This allows patient-specific sequences to be identified for the analysis of follow-up samples when used to detect subclinical and submicroscopic disease *(19,26)*, giving some confidence that what is detected is really the lymphoma-related clone and not either contamination or a translocation *de novo*.

There is some data to suggest that failure to remove t(14;18) bearing cells from autologous bone marrow harvests is associated with earlier recurrence following their use for hemopoietic rescue *(29)*, although this has not been confirmed in other studies *(19)*. Despite the uncertainty regarding the presence of translocation-bearing cells in prolonged remission, the intuitive suggestion that patients are more likely to remain disease-free if the clone is eliminated seems to be supported by some data. Patients with PCR-positive bone marrow during follow-up after myeloablative treatment have earlier recurrences *(30)*, although the relationship is less clear for peripheral blood *(31)*. The increasing use of peripheral blood progenitor cells for reconstitution after myeloablative treatment has led to studies of leukapheresis products by PCR, which has demonstrated the presence of cells bearing the translocation in most cases *(32,33)*.

For detection of the t(14;18) in lymph node biopsies or bone marrows with evidence of lymphomatous infiltration a single amplification reaction is usually adequate, but for follow-up specimens in which submicroscopic disease is sought, a "drop-in" technique followed by nested amplification improves sen-

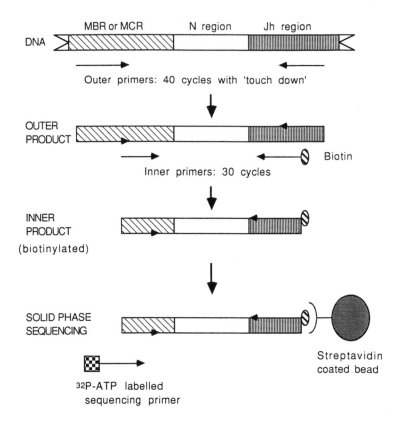

Fig. 3. Schematic representation of amplification and sequencing of t(14;18).

sitivity from 1 cell in 10^5 to between 1 in 10^6 and 10^7. The use of a biotinylated primer for one end of the final amplification allows purification of the product using streptavidin magnetic beads, which makes direct sequencing much easier to carry out in the solid phase.

The overall technique is illustrated in Fig. 3.

2. Materials

The great sensitivity of PCR requires stringent control of the laboratory in order to avoid contamination. This is a particular risk when amplified products are manipulated for sequencing, but clearly sample preparation is another stage at which this may prove a problem. The standard recommendations for avoiding false-positive results apply *(34)*.

The crucial measures to emphasize are:

1. Use of disposable plastics, rather than reusable glassware.
2. Preparation of only one biopsy or blood sample at a time.
3. Physical and temporal separation of the processes of DNA extraction, amplification, and sequencing.
4. Preparation of stocks of reaction mixtures in advance.

2.1. Tissues for Study

Successful amplification is most readily carried out using proteinase-K digests of either fresh or fresh-frozen biopsies for phenol/chloroform extraction of DNA. Paraffin-embedded sections yield less reliable DNA but the fragment size is usually adequate for PCR provided the material is not over-digested.

Blood samples and bone marrow aspirates should be prepared by density gradient centrifugation to isolate the mononuclear cell fraction. Thereafter samples may be digested directly in PCR buffer, or subjected to phenol/chloroform extraction. The latter technique risks a loss of material that may aggravate sampling error when small numbers of abnormal cells are present. Provided red cell contamination is minimized the reliability of amplification is no worse with direct digestion and PCR, which involves fewer steps and hence fewer opportunities for cross-contamination.

2.2. Solutions

Digestion and PCR buffers should be autoclaved before addition of proteinase-K. This is added fresh when samples are prepared.

1. Digestion buffer: 100 mM NaCl, 10 mM Tris-HCl, pH 8.0, 25 mM EDTA, 0.5% (v/v) SDS, and proteinase K 0.1 mg/mL for fresh or cryopreserved specimens, 0.5 mg/mL for paraffin-embedded material.
2. Phenol/chloroform/isoamyl alcohol (25:24:1).
3. Chloroform/isoamyl alcohol (24:1).
4. 3M sodium acetate, pH 5.2.
5. Absolute ethanol.
6. TE buffer: 10 mM Tris-HCl, pH 7.5 and 1 mM EDTA (autoclaved).
7. Phosphate-buffered saline: 0.02M sodium phosphate buffer and 0.127M sodium chloride, pH 7.4 (autoclaved).
8. PCR buffer: 10 mM Tris-HCl, pH 8.0, 2.5 mM MgCl$_2$, 50 mM KCl, 0.45% (v/v) Nonidet P-40, 0.45% (v/v) Tween 20 and 0.5 mg/mL proteinase K.

2.3.1. PCR Reactions

1. Deoxynucleotide triphosphates (dATP, dCTP, dGTP, dTTP), made as 10 mmol stock solutions in sterile water.
2. *Taq* polymerase and 10X reaction buffer; Mineral oil to overlay PCR tubes.
3. Oligonucleotides: All made up as 20 µmol stock solution in sterile water.
4. First stage: outer primers. Sequences are shown 5'–3', with the melting temperature indicated in the right hand column.

Outer *Bcl*-2 MBR		CAGCCTTGAAACATTGATGG	58
Outer *Bcl*-2 MCR		GACTCCTTTACGTGCTGGTACC	68
Jh consensus		ACCTGAGGAGACGGTGACC	62
Jh specific	J6	TCGGAACATGGTCCAGTCCG	64
	J5	TGCAAGCTGAGTCTCCCTAA	60
	J4	ACAAACCTCGAGTTAACGGA	58

5. Second stage (Nested PCR): inner primers.

Inner *Bcl*-2 MBR	AGTTGCTTTACGTGGCCTGT	60
Inner *Bcl*-2 MCR	GATGGCTTTGCTGAGAGGTAT	62
Jh inner consensus	CAGGGTTCCTTGGCCCCAG	64

2.4. Sequencing

1. Sephadex G-50.
2. Streptavidin-coated microbeads (Dynabeads M-280 streptavidin: Dynal, Oslo, Norway).
3. Binding buffer: 10 m*M* Tris-HCl, pH 7.5, 1 m*M* EDTA and 2.0*M* NaCl (autoclaved).
4. 0.1*M* NaOH.
5. TE buffer, pH 8.0 (autoclaved).
6. Commercial sequencing kit.

3. Methods

3.1. DNA Preparation

3.1.1. Lymph Node Biopsies

1. Cut thirty 10-μm sections and crush in 250 μL digestion buffer in a microfuge tube.
2. Incubate with proteinase K: 55°C for 1 h for fresh frozen material, and 37°C for 72 h for paraffin sections.
3. Mix with an equal volume of phenol/chloroform/isoamyl alcohol (25:24:1) and centrifuge at 14,000*g* in a microfuge for 10 min (*see* Note 1).
4. Collect the upper aqueous layer and repeat the extraction with the same mixture.
5. Collect the upper aqueous layer and extract with chloroform/isoamyl alcohol (24:1).
6. Add 1/10th vol of 3*M* sodium acetate pH 5.2 and 2 vol ethanol at –20°C.
7. Spool out the DNA precipitate on a glass rod (*see* Note 2).
8. Wash briefly in absolute ethanol.
9. Dry in air, then resuspend in 100 μL TE buffer, pH 7.5. Store at 4°C.
10. Measure concentration and purity of DNA by OD_{260} and OD_{280} (*see* Note 3).

3.1.2. Blood/Bone Marrow Aspirates

1. Layer onto an equal volume of Ficoll-hypaque 1.077 g/mL (Nycomed, Oslo, Norway) in a plastic centrifuge tube.
2. Centrifuge at 1000*g* for 25 min.

3. Remove the mononuclear cell layer from the interface.
4. Add an equal volume of phosphate-buffered saline (PBS). Centrifuge at 800*g* for 10 min.
5. Wash twice in PBS.
6. Count cells and resuspend in PCR buffer at a concentration of 5×10^6 cells/mL.
7. Incubate with proteinase K at 55°C for 1 h.
8. Denature by heating to 95°C for 5 min and store at –20°C.

3.2. PCR Reactions

3.2.1. Biopsy Specimens

Reaction mixture: DNA 1 µg for each 50 µL reaction tube.
0.2 m*M* dATP, dCTP, dGTP, dTTP   1 µL each
1 m*M* of each oligonucleotide primer   2.5 µL each
10X reaction buffer   5 µL
Sterile water to final volume of 50 µL
1 U of *Taq* polymerase added after
initial denaturation period (*see* Note 4).

Oligonucleotides: a. Outer *Bcl*-2 MBR/Jh consensus (biotinylated)
b. Outer *Bcl*-2 MCR/Jh consensus (biotinylated)

Conditions:

Denaturation	94°C	10 min	
Denaturation	94°C	45 s	Two cycles, then reducing anneal-
Annealing	60°C	1 min	ing temperature 1°C and repeating
Extension	72°C	1 min	every two cycles until 56°C
Denaturation	94°C	45 s	
Annealing	55°C	1 min	30 cycles
Extension	72°C	2 min	
Extension	72°C	5 min	

3.2.2. Follow-Up Specimens

Reaction mixture:

First (outer) stage:
DNA in PCR buffer   25 µL
0.2 m*M* dATP, dCTP, dGTP, dTTP   1 µL each
1 m*M* of each oligonucleotide primer (*see* Note 5)   2.5 µL each
10X reaction buffer   5 µL
Sterile water to final volume of 50 µL
1 U of *Taq* polymerase added after initial
denaturation period.

Second (inner) stage:

5 μL of outer stage product	
0.2 m*M* dATP, dCTP, dGTP, dTTP	1 μL each
1 μ*M* of each oligonucleotide primer	2.5 μL each
10X reaction buffer	5 μL
Sterile water to final volume of 50 μL	
1 U of *Taq* polymerase added after initial	
denaturation period.	

Oligonucleotides:

First stage:

Outer MBR or MCR *Bcl*-2 according to breakpoint previously identified.
Jh primer according to breakpoint identified on sequencing (usually J4, J5, or J6).
If no sequence data available use Jh consensus (*see* Note 6).

Second stage:

Inner MBR or MCR *Bcl*-2 according to known breakpoint.
Jh inner consensus (biotinylated).

Conditions:

Outer stage: as for biopsy specimens described (Section 3.2.1.).

Inner stage:

Denaturation	94°C	10 min	
Denaturation	94°C	45 s	
Annealing	57°C	1 min	} 30 cycles
Extension	72°C	2 min	
Extension	72°C	5 min	

All PCR products are run out on 2% agarose gels and visualized by ethidium bromide staining and UV light (*see* Note 7). The degree of sensitivity may be increased further by blotting and probing with internal oligonucleotides, although in general positive results are visible without this being necessary.

3.3. Solid-Phase Sequencing

1. Add PCR products to a Sephadex G-50 column and wash through with 50 μL TE buffer, pH 8.0 (*see* Note 8).
2. Add 40 μL of dynabeads at a concentration of 3×10^8/mL in binding buffer.
3. Allow to bind for 10 min at room temperature.
4. Pull down beads on magnet, remove supernatant, and discard.
5. Wash beads in 50 μL binding buffer. Pull down on magnet again and discard supernatant.
6. Resuspend beads in 10 μL 0.1*M* NaOH for denaturation at room temperature for 10 min.
7. Pull down beads on magnet and discard supernatant. Wash once in 50 μL 0.1*M* NaOH, once in 50 μL binding buffer and once in 50 μL TE pH 8.0.

8. Resuspend beads in sterile water according to volume required for sequencing.
9. Carry out sequencing reactions according to kit manufacturer's protocol, using inner *Bcl*-2 oligonucleotide as the sequencing primer.
10. Following termination step and addition of loading dye draw down beads on magnet and load sequencing gel with supernatant.

4. Notes

1. Following the first phenol/chloroform/isoamyl alcohol extraction there is often a viscous white layer between the aqueous and nonaqueous phases. This should not be drawn up. If pipeting is difficult owing to high viscosity the addition of further digestion buffer (without proteinase K) will dilute out the aqueous phase. If plastic pipet tips are used the excision of the narrow end with a sterile scalpel may also make it easier to draw up the viscous fluid.
2. If the DNA precipitate is not readily visible following sodium acetate/ethanol precipitation leave the mixture at –20°C overnight before centrifuging down at 10,000g. The precipitate is then washed in absolute ethanol before vacuum drying and resuspension in TE buffer.
3. Spectrophotometric determination of the amount of DNA is made by taking a reading at 260 nm. An optical density (OD) of 1 corresponds to 50 µg/mL. A further reading is taken at 280 nm and the ratio of the two readings (OD_{260}/OD_{280}) provides an estimate of the purity. A ratio above 1.8 denotes a good purity. If there is contamination with protein or phenol the ratio will fall below this value.
4. *Taq* polymerase is usually supplied with 10X reaction buffer. The concentration of magnesium may require titration to optimize the reaction. The composition of the "PCR buffer" given was determined for a particular make of *Taq* (Promega). It may require alteration according to different manufacturers' recommendations.
5. Oligonucleotide concentrations do not generally require titration with the "drop-in" technique.
6. The Jh consensus primer is adequate for amplification when relatively high copy numbers are present. However for samples containing rare translocation-bearing cells a 600 basepair artifact occurs that reduces amplification efficiency. For this reason a Jh primer specific to the patient's translocation is recommended for the first stage of amplification in follow-up specimens. The great majority of translocations occur in J4, J5, or J6.
7. MBR rearrangements give products of between 50–200 basepairs in length. MCR rearrangements give products of 500–600 basepairs. Using the Jh consensus primer may sometimes allow priming off a further segment, resulting in a second band of product 600 basepairs larger.
8. Sephadex G-50 columns are prepared by plugging the tip of a 1-mL syringe with sterile polymer wool and filling the syringe with a concentrated slurry of Sephadex made up in TE buffer. Suspend the syringe in a sterile centrifuge tube and spin at 800g for 3 min. Discard the centrifuge tube and place the syringe in a clean one. Add the PCR product to the top of the column with 50 µL of TE buffer and spin down again at 800g for 3 min. Collect the eluted product from the bottom of the tube.

References

1. Fukuhara, S. and Rowley, J. D. (1978) Chromosome 14 translocations in non-Burkitt lymphomas. *Int. J. Cancer* **22**, 14–21.
2. Yunis, J. J., Oken, M. M., Kaplan, M. E., Ensrud, K. M., Hore, R. R., and Theologides, A. (1982) Distinctive chromosomal abnormalities in histologic subtypes of non-Hodgkin's lymphoma. *N. Engl. J. Med.* **307**, 1231–1236.
3. Bloomfield, C. D., Arthur, D. C., Frizzera, G., Levine, E. G., Peterson, B. A., and Gajl-Peczalska, K. J. (1983) Nonrandom chromosome abnormalities in lymphoma. *Cancer Res.* **43**, 2975–2984.
4. Rowley, J. D. (1988) Chromosome studies in non-Hodgkin's lymphomas: The role of the 14;18 translocation. *J. Clin. Oncol.* **6**, 919–925.
5. Tsujimoto, Y., Gorham, J., Cossman, J., Jaffe, E., and Croce, C. (1985) The t(14;18) chromosome translocations involved in B-cell neoplasms result from mistakes in VDJ joining. *Science* **229**, 1390–1393.
6. Cleary, M. L. and Sklar, J. (1985) Nucleotide sequence of a t(14;18) chromosomal breakpoint in follicular lymphoma and demonstration of a breakpoint cluster region near a transcriptionally active locus on chromosome 18. *Proc. Natl. Acad. Sci. USA* **82**, 7439–7443.
7. Chen-Levy, Z., Nourse, J., and Cleary, M. L. (1989) The *Bcl*-2 candidate proto-oncogene product is a 24-kilodalton integral-membrane protein highly expressed in lymphoid cell lines and lymphomas carrying the t(14;18) translocation. *Mol. Cell. Biol.* **9**, 701–10.
8. Ngan, B. Y., Chen-Levy, Z., Weiss, L. M., Warnke, R. A., and Cleary, M. L. (1988) Expression in non-Hodgkin's lymphoma of the *Bcl*-2 protein associated with the t(14;18) chromosomal translocation. *N. Engl. J. Med.* **318**, 1638–1644.
9. Hockenberry, D., Nunez, G., Milliman, C., Schreiber, R. D., and Korsmeyer, S. J. (1990) *BCL*-2 is an inner mitochondrial membrane protein that blocks programmed cell death. *Nature* **348**, 334–336.
10. Liu, Y.-J., Mason, D. Y., Johnson, G. D., Abbot, S., Gregory, C. D., Hardie, D. L., Gordon, J., and MacLennan, I. C. M. (1991) Germinal center cells express *Bcl*-2 protein after activation by signals which prevent their entry into apoptosis. *Eur. J. Immunol.* **21**, 1905–1910.
11. Silverman, G. A., Green, E. D., Young, R. L., Jockel, J. I., Domer, P. H., and Korsmeyer, S. J. (1990) Meiotic recombination between yeast artificial chromosomes yields a single clone containing the entire *Bcl*-2 proto-oncogene. *Proc. Natl. Acad. Sci. USA* **87**, 9913–9917.
12. Cleary, M. L., Galili, N., and Sklar, J. (1986) Detection of a second t(14;18) breakpoint cluster region in human follicular lymphomas. *J. Exp. Med.* **164**, 315–320.
13. Tanaka, S., Louie, D. C., Kant, J. A., and Reed, J. C. (1992) Frequent incidence of somatic mutations in translocated *BCL*-2 oncogenes of non-Hodgkin's lymphomas. *Blood* **79**, 229–237.
14. Lee, M. S., Chang, K. S., Cabanillas, F., Freireich, E. J., Trujillo, J. M., and Stass, S. A. (1987) Detection of minimal residual cells carrying the t(14;18) by DNA sequence amplification. *Science* **237**, 175–178.

15. Crescenzi, M., Seto, M., Herzig, G. P., Weiss, P. D., Griffith, R. C., and Korsmeyer, S. J. (1988) Thermostable DNA polymerase chain amplification of t(14;18) chromosome breakpoints and detection of minimal residual disease. *Proc. Natl. Acad. Sci. USA* **85,** 4869–4873.

16. Ngan, B. Y., Nourse, J., and Cleary, M. L. (1989) Detection of chromosomal translocation t(14;18) within the minor cluster region of *Bcl-2* by polymerase chain reaction and direct genomic sequencing of the enzymatically amplified DNA in follicular lymphomas. *Blood* **73,** 1759–1762.

17. Cotter, F., Price, C., Zucca, E., and Young, B. D. (1990) Direct sequence analysis of the 14q+ and 18q- chromosome junctions in follicular lymphoma. *Blood* **76,** 131–135.

18. Bakshi, A., Wright, J. J., Graninger, W., Seto, M., Owens, J., Cossman, J., Jensen, J. P., Goldman, P., and Korsmeyer, S. J. (1987) Mechanism of the t(14;18) chromosomal translocation: structural analysis of both derivative 14 and 18 reciprocal partners. *Proc. Natl. Acad. Sci. USA* **84,** 2396–2400.

19. Johnson, P. W. M., Price, C. G. A., Smith, T., Cotter, F. E., Meerabux, J., Rohatiner, A. Z. S., Young, B. D., and Lister, T. A. (1994) Detection of cells bearing the t(14;18) translocation following myeloablative treatment and autologous bone marrow transplantation for follicular lymphoma. *J. Clin. Oncol.* **12,** 798–805.

20. Aisenberg, A. C., Wilkes, B. M., and Jacobson, J. O. (1988) The *Bcl-2* gene is rearranged in many diffuse B-cell lymphomas. *Blood* **71,** 969–72.

21. Stetler-Stevenson, M., Crush-Stanton, S., and Cossman, J. (1990) Involvement of the *Bcl-2* gene in Hodgkin's disease. *J. Nat. Cancer Inst.* **82,** 855.

22. Gupta, R. K., Whelan, J. S., Lister, T. A., Young, B. D., and Bodmer, J. G. (1992) Direct sequence analysis of the t(14;18) chromosomal translocation in Hodgkin's disease. *Blood* **79,** 2084–2088.

23. Limpens, J., de Jong, D., van Krieken, J. H., Price, C. G., Young, B. D., van Ommen, G. J., et al. (1991) *Bcl-2/JH* rearrangements in benign lymphoid tissues with follicular hyperplasia. *Oncogene* **6,** 2271–2276.

24. Aster, J. C., Kobayashi, Y., Shiota, M., Mori, S., and Sklar, J. (1992) Detection of the t(14;18) at similar frequencies in hyperplastic lymphoid tissues from American and Japanese patients. *Am. J. Path.* **141,** 291–299.

25 Limpens, J., Stad, R., de Vlaam, C., Schuuring, E., van Krieken, J. H., and Kluin, P. M. (1992) B-cells with the lymphoma associated translocation t(14;18) are present in the blood B-cells of normal individuals. *Blood* **80(Suppl 1),** 258a.

26. Price, C. G. A., Meerabux, J., Murtagh, S., Cotter, F. E., Rohatiner, A. Z. S., Young, B. D., and Lister, T. A. (1991) The significance of circulating cells carrying t(14;18) in long remission from follicular lymphoma. *J. Clin. Oncol.* **9,** 1527–1532.

27. Finke, J., Slanina, J., Lange, W., and Dolken, G. (1993) Persistence of circulating t(14;18)-positive cells in long-term remission after radiation therapy for localized-stage follicular lymphoma. *J. Clin. Oncol.* **11,** 1668–1673.

28. Lambrechts, A. C., Hupkes, P. E., Dorssers, L. C. J., and van't Veer, M. B. (1994) Clinical significance of t(14;18)-positive cells in the circulation of patients with stage III or IV follicular non-Hodgkin's lymphoma during first remission. *J. Clin. Oncol.* **12,** 1541–1546.

29. Gribben, J. G., Freedman, A. S., Neuberg, D., Roy, D. C., Blake, K. W., Woo, S. D., Grossbard, M. L., Rabinowe, S. N., Coral, F., Freeman, G. J., Ritz, J., and Nadler, L. M. (1991) Immunologic purging of marrow assessed by PCR before autologous bone marrow transplantation for B-cell lymphoma. *N. Engl. J. Med.* **325,** 1525–1533.

30. Gribben, J. G., Neuberg, D., Freedman, A. S., Gimmi, C. D., Pesek, K. W., Barber, M., Saporito, L., Woo, S. D., Coral, F., and Spector, N. (1993) Detection by polymerase chain-reaction of residual cells with the *Bcl*-2 translocation is associated with increased risk of relapse after autologous bone-marrow transplantation for b-cell lymphoma. *Blood* **81,** 3449–3457.

31. Gribben, J. G., Neuberg, D., Barber, M., Moore, J., Pesek, K. W., Freedman, A. S., and Nadler, L. W. (1994) Detection of residual lymphoma-cells by polymerase chain-reaction in peripheral-blood is significantly less predictive for relapse than detection in bone-marrow. *Blood* **83,** 3800–3807.

32. Haas, R., Moos, M., Karcher, A., Mohle, R., Witt, B., Goldschmidt, H., Fruhauf, S., Flentje, M., Wannenmacher, M., and Hunstein, W. (1994) Sequential high-dose therapy with peripheral-blood progenitor-cell support in low-grade non-Hodgkin's lymphoma. *J. Clin. Oncol.* **12,** 1685–1692.

33. Negrin, R. S. and Pesando, J. (1994) Detection of tumor cells in purged bone marrow and peripheral-blood mononuclear cells by polymerase chain reaction amplification of *Bcl*-2 translocations. *J. Clin. Oncol.* **12,** 1021–1027.

34. Kwok, S. and Higuchi, R. (1989) Avoiding false positives with PCR. *Nature* **339,** 237–238.

Further Reading

Erlich, H. A. (1991) *PCR Technology,* Stockton Press, New York.

Innis, M. A., Gelfand, D. H., Sninsky, J. J., and White, T. J. (1992) *PCR Protocols,* Academic, San Diego.

Lemoine, N. R. and Wright, N. A. (1993) *The Molecular Pathology of Cancer. Cancer Surveys,* vol. 16. Cold Spring Harbor Laboratory Press, Cold Spring Harbor, NY.

7

NPM-ALK Reverse Transcriptase-Polymerase Chain Reaction Analysis for Detection of the t(2;5) Translocation of Non-Hodgkin's Lymphoma

Sheila A. Shurtleff, James R. Downing, and Stephan W. Morris

1. Introduction

The diagnosis and classification of non-Hodgkin's lymphoma (NHL) has traditionally been made based on morphologic and immunophenotypic criteria. Unfortunately, because of the diverse nature of this group of diseases, reliance solely on these criteria has frequently resulted in misdiagnosis. In addition, investigators have been limited in their ability to define biologically and clinically relevant non-Hodgkin's lymphoma subgroups using this diagnostic approach. The development of modern molecular biological techniques and their use to characterize the genetic abnormalities that are of pathogenic significance in NHL now provides an additional means to identify and to rationally subcategorize these neoplasms. The shortcomings of traditional methods of NHL diagnosis and classification have been especially evident within the morphological subset commonly referred to as the large-cell lymphomas, which comprise approx 25 and 40% of NHL in children and adults, respectively (1). The marked cytological, immunological, and clinical heterogeneity of this group of tumors suggests that it is comprised of several biologically different neoplasms. However, morphological and immunophenotypic subclassification of the large-cell lymphomas has failed to identify a subset of tumors having a reproducibly different therapeutic response or patient survival rate. Until recently, recurrent genetic abnormalities characteristic of the large-cell lymphomas had not been identified. However, the characterization during the

From: *Methods in Molecular Medicine, Molecular Diagnosis of Cancer*
Edited by: F. E. Cotter Humana Press Inc., Totowa, NJ

past 2 yr of chromosomal rearrangements involving the *BCL6/LAZ3* zinc finger gene located at 3q27 (which is altered in approx 30% of these tumors *[2,3])*, and the cloning by our group *(4)* of the *NPM-ALK* fusion gene produced by the t(2;5) may now permit the identification of molecular genetic subtypes of large-cell lymphoma that possess unique biological and/or clinical features.

The t(2;5)(p23;q35) was originally identified as a recurrent cytogenetic abnormality in cases of anaplastic large-cell lymphoma (ALCL) that express the Ki-1 (CD30) antigen, a cytokine receptor for a ligand related to the tumor necrosis factor family *(5)*. Because of their anaplastic features, these tumors, which are primarily of T-cell lineage (75%), are frequently misdiagnosed as other conditions including Hodgkin's disease, malignant histiocytosis, mycosis fungoides, poorly differentiated carcinoma metastatic to lymph nodes, or even viral infections. Clinically, Ki-1+ lymphomas/ALCL are aggressive tumors that produce frequent extranodal disease involving skin, bone, soft tissue, gastrointestinal tract, and/or lung and that exhibit a bimodal age distribution similar to that observed in Hodgkin's disease *(6)*. Despite the historical association of the t(2;5) with Ki-1+ lymphomas/ALCL, molecular studies performed using the reverse transcriptase-polymerase chain reaction (RT-PCR) methods described here indicate that the translocation also occurs in a significant fraction of large-cell lymphomas with immunoblastic or diffuse morphology *(7)*. Moreover, only slightly more than half of the cases with anaplastic morphology and slightly less than two-thirds of the Ki-1+ cases analyzed in these studies contained the t(2;5). Thus, this molecular genetic subtype of NHL occurs in all morphologic types of large-cell lymphoma and is present independent of Ki-1 antigen status. Overall, based upon the clinical cytogenetic literature, approx 25% of large-cell lymphomas (or about 10% of all NHL) contain the t(2;5). Confirmation of this frequency of occurrence, as well as the determination of whether this molecularly-defined subtype of lymphoma constitutes a distinct subtype prognostically and/or therapeutically, presently await the analysis of large, unselected NHL treatment groups.

Using a positional cloning approach, we recently cloned the t(2;5), demonstrating it to involve the genes encoding nucleophosmin (*NPM*), a nucleolar phosphoprotein on chromosome 5, and a novel receptor tyrosine kinase, anaplastic lymphoma kinase (*ALK*), on chromosome 2 *(4)*. The translocation results in a chimeric *NPM-ALK* fusion gene and transcript that is encoded on the der(5) chromosome, and produces a fusion protein consisting of the amino-terminal portion of *NPM* fused in-frame to the kinase domain of *ALK* (*see* Fig. 1). *NPM* is a highly conserved (ubiquitously expressed) 38-kDa nonribosomal RNA-binding protein that shuttles ribosomal ribonucleoproteins between the nucleolus and the cytoplasm and is involved in the late stages of preribosomal particle assembly *(8,9)*. *ALK* is a member of the insulin receptor subfamily,

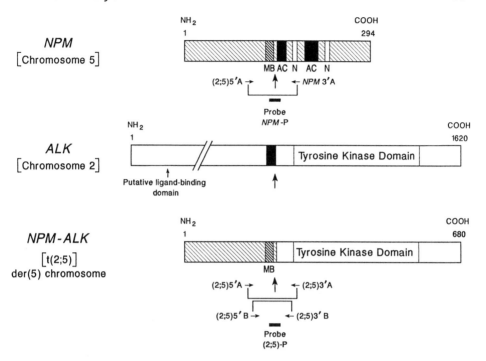

Fig. 1. Schematic representation of the proteins encoded by the normal *NPM* and *ALK* genes and by the *NPM-ALK* fusion gene derived from the derivative 5 chromosome that is produced by the t(2;5). NPM is a ubiquitously expressed nucleolar phosphoprotein that normally functions as a shuttle protein for ribonucleoproteins from the nucleolus to the ribosomes in the cytoplasm *(8)*. The metal binding (MB), acidic amino acid clusters (AC), and nuclear localization signals (N) of NPM are indicated *(9)*. ALK is a newly described receptor tyrosine kinase of the insulin receptor subfamily *(4)*. The presumed ligand-binding, transmembrane (TM), and intracytoplasmic kinase catalytic domains of ALK are shown. The positions at which the fusion junctions occur in the t(2;5) translocation are indicated by arrows. The der(5)-derived *NPM-ALK* chimeric gene produces a 75-kDa product consisting of the amino-terminal portion of NPM fused to the cytoplasmic domain of ALK. The approximate position of the oligonucleotide primers and probes used for RT-PCR analysis of the t(2;5) are indicated.

having greatest homology to leukocyte tyrosine kinase (*LTK*) *(4)*. The ligand(s) that bind ALK and the normal functions of this receptor tyrosine kinase are presently unknown. As a result of the t(2;5), transcription of the portion of the *ALK* gene encoding its kinase domain is driven by the strong *NPM* gene promoter, leading to its inappropriate expression in lymphoid cells (in which *ALK* is usually transcriptionally silent). Furthermore, as a result of its fusion with *NPM*, the *ALK* kinase domain is constitutively activated and is relocalized from its normal position at the outer cellular membrane to within both the cytoplasm and nucleus of lymphoma cells; the oncogenic ability of the chimeric NPM-ALK protein can be readily demonstrated by in vitro transformation assays using immortalized rodent fibroblast lines such as NIH-3T3 (S.W. Morris, unpublished observations).

Our characterization of the t(2;5) has permitted the development of an RT-PCR assay using primers derived from *NPM* and *ALK* sequences bracketing the *NPM-ALK* fusion junction that allows rapid and sensitive detection of the translocation in clinical material. We have used this assay to successfully detect *NPM-ALK* transcripts in 28 of 29 cases of NHL known to contain the t(2;5) by cytogenetic analysis and in 10 of 48 cases that either lacked this cytogenetic abnormality or had unsuccessful cytogenetics *(4,7)*. Thus, the RT-PCR assay described here should permit the detection of the t(2;5)-derived *NPM-ALK* fusion gene in the vast majority of cases containing this translocation.

A brief mention regarding the use of the RT-PCR assay described here in the analysis of suspected Hodgkin's disease is warranted. An area of controversy that has existed for some time has been the biological relationship between Ki-1+ lymphoma/ALCL and Hodgkin's disease *(10)*. Although a morphologic distinction can be made in most situations, there exist cases in which the pathologic distinction is ill-defined. Moreover, so-called "secondary ALCL" has been noted to develop either simultaneously with or subsequent to Hodgkin's disease. In addition, both ALCL and the malignant Reed-Sternberg cells of Hodgkin's disease strongly express the Ki-1 antigen. Thus, whether these two lymphomas represent morphologic variants of a single biologic disease or constitute separate entities has been and remains a point of controversy. In light of the uncertain relationship between these neoplasms, the development of a sensitive RT-PCR assay for detection of the t(2;5) has prompted a number of groups to examine Hodgkin's disease cases for the presence of the translocation. To date, in four independent studies (summarized in refs. *11* and *12*), 129 Hodgkin's disease patients with tumors of all histological subtypes have been analyzed and found to lack evidence of the t(2;5). By contrast, a single small study has reported RT-PCR detection of the t(2;5) in 11 of 13 patients with Hodgkin's disease *(13)*. The reason for the striking difference between these studies is presently unclear, and resolution of this issue will require the analysis of additional patients. However, given that the great majority of patients analyzed in studies to date have been found to be t(2;5)-negative, combined with the fact that the translocation has never been observed in cytogenetic studies of Hodgkin's disease *(14,15)*, it is most likely that the t(2;5) is rarely, if ever, found in Hodgkin's disease and that RT-PCR analysis will be useful in distinguishing Ki-1+ non-Hodgkin's lymphoma from Hodgkin's disease.

2. Solutions and Materials

2.1. RNA Extraction

There are a number of methods that can be used for RNA extraction. We are currently using Purescript RNA isolation kits from Gentra Systems (Research Triangle Park, NC). If appropriate kits are unavailable, the procedure outlined here works well. It uses a lysing solution containing guanidinium thiocyanate to inactivate RNases, followed by a number of extractions *(16)*. This method gives a reasonable yield (10–20 μg) of RNA that is relatively free from contaminating DNA from 1×10^7 starting cells. Any other method of extraction that gives comparable quality RNA can be used.

2.1.1. Solutions Required for RNA Extraction

1. Diethylpyrocarbonate (DEPC)-treated water: Add 200 μL of DEPC (Sigma, St. Louis, MO) to 1 L of water. Shake well, then loosen cap and incubate for 2–8 h at 37°C. Autoclave, then shake again to remove DEPC breakdown products.
2. 10% Sarcosine: Add 250 mL of DEPC-treated water to 25 g of N-lauroyl sarcosine (Sigma), filter through a 0.45-μ sterile filter system, and store at room temperature.
3. 0.75M Citric acid: Add 400 mL of DEPC-treated H_2O to 78.75 g of citric acid (Sigma), then bring volume up to 500 mL.
4. 0.75M Sodium citrate, pH 7.0: Add 400 mL of DEPC-treated H_2O to 110 g of sodium citrate (Sigma), pH to 7.0 with 0.75M citric acid, then make up to 500 mL.
5. Denaturing solution: 4M guanidinium thiocyanate, 25 mM sodium citrate, pH 7.0; 0.5% sarcosine. Add 117.2 mL of DEPC-treated water to a 100-g bottle of guanidinium thiocyanate (Fluka Chemicals, Ron Konkoma, NY), then add 10.5 mL of 10% sarcosine, 7.04 mL of 0.75M sodium citrate, pH 7.0, swirl container to mix, and heat at 65°C to aid in dissolution if necessary.
6. Solution "D": Add 360 μL of β-mercaptoethanol (Sigma) to 50 mL of denaturing solution. This solution should be aliquoted and can be stored for 1 mo at room temperature.
7. Phenol (water-saturated), pH 6.6 (Amresco, Solon, OH). Store at 4°C.
8. Chloroform (Fisher, Pittsburgh, PA): Store at room temperature in a dark bottle.
9. Isoamyl alcohol (Sigma): Store at room temperature.
10. Chloroform/isoamyl alcohol: Add 4 mL of isoamyl alcohol to 96 mL of chloroform. Store at room temperature in a dark bottle.
11. Isopropanol (Fisher): Store at room temperature.
12. 75% Ethanol: Add 25 mL of DEPC-treated water to 75 mL of absolute ethanol (Aaper, Shelbyville, KY).
13. Glacial acetic acid (Fisher): Store at room temperature.
14. 2M Sodium acetate (NaOAc, Fisher), pH 4.0. Add 15 mL of DEPC-treated water to 136 g of sodium acetate, add glacial acetic acid until pH is 4.0, then make up to 500 mL. Store at room temperature.
15. RNasin (Promega, Madison, WI): 40 U/mL. Store at 20°C.

2.1.2. Materials Required for RNA Extraction

1. Labconco RNA isolation hood (optional): Model 5102 (Labconco, Kansas City, MO).
2. Pipetors: P1000, P200, P20 (Rainin, Woburn, MA).
3. 1.7 mL siliconized microfuge tubes (PGC Scientific, Frederick, MD).
4. SpeedVac (Savant, Farmingdale, NY).
5. Water bath (Fisher), set at 37°C.
6. Eppendorf microfuge (Brinkman Instruments, Westbury, NY).

2.2. RT-PCR of the t(2;5)

2.2.1. Solutions for RT-PCR of the t(2;5)

1. Oligonucleotides (required for primer extension):

    (2;5)5'A, 5'-GCTTTGAAATAACACCACCAG-3', 5' oligo for t(2;5).
    (2;5)3'A, 5'-TAGTTGGGGTTGTAGTCGGT-3', 3' oligo for t(2;5).
    (2;5)5'B, 5'-CCAGTGGTCTTAAGGTTG-3', 5' nesting oligo for t(2;5).
    (2;5)3'B, 5'-TACTCAGGGCTCTGCAGC-3', 3' nesting oligo for t(2;5).
    (2;5)5'A, same as above, 5' oligo for *NPM* control.
    *NPM*3'A, 5'-CAGACCGCTTTCCAGATATAC-3', 3' oligo for *NPM* control.
    (2,5)-P, 5'-AGCACTTAGTAGTGTACCGCCGGA-3', probe for t(2;5).
    NPM-P, 5'-GTGCTGTCCACTAATATGCAC-3', probe for *NPM* control.

    Primers (2;5)5'A and (2;5)3'A are used to amplify the t(2;5)-derived *NPM-ALK* fusion gene transcripts and generate a 177-bp product. Primers (2;5)5'A and *NPM* 3'A are used as a positive control to detect *NPM* gene transcripts, which are ubiquitously expressed at high levels, in order to check the quality of the RNA. This primer pair generates a 185-bp *NPM* PCR product. Primers (2;5)5'B and (2;5)3'B are nesting oligos that can be used to further amplify the t(2;5) PCR fusion product for increased sensitivity of detection, if necessary. This primer pair generates a 123-bp *NPM-ALK* product. Probe (2;5)-P is a junction specific probe to detect the *NPM-ALK* fusion product. Probe *NPM*-P is used to detect the control *NPM* PCR product. Store at –20°C.

2. DMSO (dimethyl sulfoxide, Sigma): *See* Note 1—Stored at room temperature.
3. dNTPs (deoxynucleotide triphosphates, Perkin-Elmer Cetus, Norwalk, CT). A stock dNTP solution is made which is 1.25 mM with respect to each dNTP for both cDNA production and PCR amplification. Store at –70°C.
4. DTT (dithiothreitol, Gibco, Grand Island, NY): *See* Note 2—The stock solution is 0.1M and is stored at –70°C.
5. DEPC-treated H$_2$O. (*See* Section 2.1.1.)
6. PCR buffer: 10X by Perkin-Elmer Cetus (100 mM Tris-HCl, pH 8.3, 500 mM KCl, 15 mM MgC1$_2$, 0.01% gelatin); 5X buffer by Invitrogen (San Diego, CA); 300 mM Tris-HCl, pH 9.0; 75 mM (NH$_4$)$_2$SO$_4$, 10 mM MgCl$_2$. Both buffers are stored at –70°C.
7. Reverse transcriptase (RT): Stock is Moloney Murine Leukemia Virus RT (Life Technologies, Grand Island, NY) at a concentration of 200 U/μL. Store at –20°C.
8. RNasin: *See* Note 3—Stock is 40 U/μL (Promega). Store at –20°C.
9. *Taq* DNA polymerase: Stock is 5 U/μL (Perkin-Elmer Cetus). Store at –20°C.

2.2.2. Materials for RT-PCR of the t(2;5)

1. Thermocycler (Perkin-Elmer Cetus 9600 or 480).
2. Eppendorf microcentrifuge.
3. 37°C Water bath.
4. 95°C Heating block (Equatherm, Melrose Park, IL).
5. Sterile hood (optional but desirable) (Baker, Sanford, ME).
6. Gloves.
7. Microfuge tubes—siliconized.
8. Aerosol resistant barrier pipet tips (ART tips, Molecular Bioproducts, San Diego, CA).
9. Pipetors.
10. Ice trays.

2.3. Solutions and Materials for Gel Electrophoresis and Southern Analysis

1. 10X Tris borate electrophoresis buffer (TBE): 108 g Tris base, 55 g boric acid, and 40 mL of 0.5M EDTA. Made up to 1 L and autoclaved. Store at room temperature.
2. 6X loading buffer: 0.25% xylene cyanol, 0.25% bromophenol blue, and 30% glycerol.
3. Ethidium bromide: Stock 10 mg/mL, final concentration 10 μg/mL in 1X TBE.
4. Agarose.
5. Nylon or nitrocellulose hybridization membranes.
6. 20X SSC stock solution: 3M sodium chloride, 1M sodium citrate.
7. 20% SDS stock solution: 20 g of SDS in 100 mL of water. Wear a mask when making this up and gently heat to dissolve, but do not boil.
8. (2;5)-P oligonucleotide primer (1 μM stock).
9. Paper towels.
10. 10X T4 end-labeling buffer (manufacturer's specification).
11. T4 polynucleotide kinase (10 U/reaction).
12. $\gamma^{32}P$ dATP (specific activity >3000 Ci/mmol).
13. Distilled water.
14. X-ray film.

3. Methods

3.1. RNA Extraction

3.1.1. General Considerations

Since RNA is easily degraded, extreme care should be taken when handling samples (*see* Notes 4 and 5). Ideally, RNA should be extracted in an area dedicated solely for that purpose and away from areas used for cloning and DNA work (*see* Note 6). Gloves should be worn at all times and work areas and instruments decontaminated with bleach or ultra violet irradiation. All solutions, with the exception of Tris, should be treated with the RNase inhibitor DEPC. Solutions are treated 2–8 h with 0.1% DEPC at 37°C, followed by autoclaving as described in Section 2.1.1. Tris solutions should be made with DEPC-autoclaved water. Sterile disposable plasticware should be used whenever possible; all glassware used should be DEPC-treated.

Stock reagents required for RNA extraction should be prepared in volumes small enough to use completely within a relatively short period (1–2 mo) since reagents such as phenol, "solution D," and chloroform have a limited shelf life. It is also desirable to limit the number of times one enters the same reagent bottle to decrease the possibility of sample crosscontamination. Owing to the extreme sensitivity of RT-PCR (allowing the detection of one abnormal cell in 100,000 cells in the case of the assay described here), it is necessary to take every precaution to reduce the risk of crosscontamination of samples. With this goal in mind, oligos and reagents used for either the reverse transcription (RT) reaction or the PCR should be aliquoted to single run volumes so that a vial is thawed, used, and then discarded. Separate sets of pipetors should be dedicated for RNA extraction, RT-PCR amplification, and postamplification analysis. The lab should have dedicated areas, or ideally separate rooms, designated for RNA extraction, RT-PCR amplification, and postamplification analysis. Large RNA extractions from positive or negative control samples should be done in a separate area away from patient RNA extractions. Under no circumstances should PCR product be brought back into the area where RT-PCR is set up.

3.1.2. Specific Procedures

1. Aliquot 400 µL of Solution "D" into 1.7-mL microfuge tubes, add 2 µg of glycogen and label tubes with pertinent information (patient name, ID number, date, and so on). In addition to the patient samples, one tube is needed for a negative extraction control (no cells added to this tube), one tube for a negative cell line control (e.g., HL-60) (17), and one tube for a positive cell line control (a t[2;5]-positive lymphoma cell line such as SU-DHL-1) (18).
2. To each tube add $1–2 \times 10^7$ cells.
3. Quick spin for 1 s at 2000g in a microcentrifuge.
4. Add 40 µL of 2M NaOAc to each sample. Close lid and flick to mix.
5. Add 400 µL of water-saturated phenol to each tube. Close lid and flick to mix.
6. Add 82 µL chloroform/isoamyl alcohol (24:1) to each tube.
7. Vortex each tube for 10 s, then place on ice for 15 min.
8. Centrifuge all samples at 16,000g for 20 min at 4°C.
9. Transfer the top aqueous phase to a new 1.7-mL microfuge tube and place on ice. (Be careful not to remove any of the organic phase or white interface.)

10. Add an equal volume of isopropanol to the aqueous layer of each sample.
11. Vortex each sample for 5 s, and place on dry ice for 30 min (or at $-70°C$ overnight).
12. Centrifuge samples at $16,000g$ for 15 min at $4°C$.
13. Remove the supernatant from each sample, taking care not to disturb the small white RNA pellet on the bottom and side wall of the tube.
14. SpeedVac each sample until dry.
15. Resuspend pellets in 300 of Solution "D," making sure pellet is completely dissolved.
16. Add 300 µL of isopropanol to each sample.
17. Vortex each sample for 5 s, then quick spin by microfuging at $2000g$ for 1–2 s.
18. Place each sample on dry ice for 30 min (or overnight at $-70°C$).
19. Centrifuge each sample at $16,000g$ for 10 min at $4°C$.
20. Remove the supernatant from each sample, taking care not to disturb the small white RNA pellet on the bottom side wall.
21. Add 500 µL of chilled 75% ethanol to each sample.
22. Vortex each sample until pellet is dislodged from the bottom of the microfuge tube.
23. Centrifuge each sample at $16,000g$ for 10 min at $4°C$.
24. Carefully remove the supernatant from each sample without disturbing the RNA pellet.
25. Speed vac each sample for 10 min (pellets should appear dry).
26. Resuspend pellets in 10 µL DEPC-water and add 1 µL RNasin.
27. Vortex each sample several times to dissolve RNA, then quick spin.
28. Store samples frozen at $-70°C$.

3.2. RT-PCR

3.2.1. Controls

Each RT-RCR will typically include the reverse transcription and amplification of RNA extractions from several patients and controls. As mentioned in the RNA extraction procedure, several negative and positive controls are used, which include the following:

1. A negative RNA control. This is a tube that had no cells added prior to the extraction that is used to ensure that all of the RNA extraction solutions are free of contaminating nucleic acids.
2. An HL-60 (or comparable cell line) negative RNA control. A cell line, such as HL-60, that does not contain the t(2;5) translocation, should also be included as a negative control *(17)*. RT-PCR of RNA from such a cell line should be positive for the control product (from the normal *NPM* gene) but negative for the t(2;5) *NPM-ALK* fusion product. If this sample is positive for the t(2;5), it indicates that contamination occurred during the run and makes all other results uninterpretable.
3. A positive SU-DHL-1 RNA control. The SU-DHL-1 lymphoma cell line contains the t(2;5) *(18)*. Therefore, RT-PCR of RNA from this cell line should be positive for both the *NPM* control and the t(2;5)-derived *NPM-ALK* product. If no *NPM-ALK* signal is present, it indicates that a reagent used, often an oligo, was not good and renders all other results uninterpretable. Again, owing to the

extreme sensitivity of RT-PCR, a number of precautions should be taken to eliminate possible sources of contamination. All stocks of reagents, with the possible exception of enzymes, should be in single-run aliquots. The RT-PCR must be set up in a hood, in a separate room or area, which can be ultra-violet light sterilized between runs. Disposable isolation gowns and gloves should be worn during RT-PCR and all reagents needed should be brought on wet or dry ice so that once the RT-PCR run is started, it is not necessary to leave the hood area until the samples are ready to go into the thermocycler. If it becomes necessary to leave, a new pair of gloves and gown should be put on upon re-entry.

3.2.2. RT Reaction

Each RT run should include separate tubes for each patient sample, a "No RNA" negative control, a negative control cell line RNA, and a positive cell line RNA. RT is done in a 20-µL total volume. If possible, all of the following steps should be done in a sterile hood.

1. Label two 1.7-mL centrifuge tubes, one for the t(2;5) and one for the *NPM* control.
2. Add the following amounts of each reagent to the tubes **for each sample and control to be analyzed:**

RT Mixes		Final conc. (in 20 µL)
10X PCR buffer (Perkin-Elmer Cetus)	2 µL/reaction	1X
dNTPs (1.25 m*M* stock)	2 µL/reaction	0.125 m*M*
DTT (0.1*M* stock)	2 µL/reaction	10 m*M*
oligo (2;5)3'A for t(2;5) mix **or** oligo *NPM* 3'A for *NPM* control (use 10 pmol of the appropriate oligo per run)		0.5 pmol/µL
RNasin (40 U/µL)	0.5µL/reaction	1 U/µL
Reverse transcriptase (200 U/µL)	1 µL/reaction	10 U/µL
DEPC-treated water	Make up to 9 µL/reaction	

3. Label 0.5-mL microfuge tubes, two for each patient and controls. Aliquot patient and control RNAs (0.5–1 µL of total RNA from each sample) into appropriate tubes and make up to 11 µL. Heat at 95°C for 5 min. (Remember to set up for two PCR runs: one for the t(2;5) and one for the *NPM* control.)
4. Quick spin samples in microcentrifuge, then set on ice.
5. Add 9 µL of either the t(2;5) or *NPM*-RT mix (Section 3.2.2., step 2) to each RNA tube (*see* Note 7).
6. Incubate in a 37°C water bath for 1 h.

3.2.3. PCR Reaction

While the RNA is being reverse transcribed, the PCR oligo mixes can be set up. Alternately, the PCR oligo mixes can be made at the same time as the RT mixes with the exception of the *Taq* polymerase enzyme, which should be added just prior to use. PCR mixes are made up in a total volume of 80 μL/reaction; this volume is added to each 20 μL vol of cDNA following RT.

1. Make up:

Oligo mix for t(2;5)		Final concentration
Oligos (2;5)5'A and (2;5)3'A	0.075 μg of each per reaction	0.10–0.15 μM
5X Buffer (pH 9.0) (Invitrogen)	16 μL/reaction	1X
DMSO	5 μL/reaction	5%
Taq polymerase (5 U/μL)	0.5 μL/reaction	0.025 U/μL
DEPC-H$_2$O	Make up to 80 μL/reaction	

Oligo mix for *NPM* controls		Final concentration
Oligos (2;5)5'A and *NPM* 3'A	0.075 μg of each per reaction	0.10–0.15 μM
10X Buffer (Perkin-Elmer Cetus)	8 μL/reaction	1X
Taq polymerase (5 U/μL)	0.5 μL/reaction	0.025 U/μL
DEPC-H$_2$O	Make up to 80 μL/reaction	

2. If the *NPM-ALK* fusion product is barely detectable or absent, a nesting PCR reaction can be run using 5% of the reaction mix from the first run. This starting volume is brought up to 20 μL, then 80 μL of the nesting oligo mix is added.

Nesting oligo mix		Final concentration
Oligos (2;5)5'B and (2;5)3'B	0.075 μg of each per reaction	0.10–0.15 μM
dNTPs (1.25 m*M* stock)	2 μL/reaction	25 μM
10X Buffer (Perkin-Elmer Cetus)	8 μL/reaction	1X
DMSO	5 μL/reaction	5%
Taq polymerase (5 U/μL)	0.5 μL/reaction	0.025 U/μL
DEPC-H$_2$O	Make up to 80 μL/reaction	

3. Samples are overlaid with one drop of mineral oil unless the run is done in a Perkin-Elmer Cetus 9600 PCR machine, in which case oil is not needed. A 62°C

annealing temperature should be used regardless of which thermocycler is used. Two examples of programs for two different machines are given below.

Bios Thermocycler (Bios Corporation, New Haven, CT):

Cycle/step	Temperature	Time
1/1	94°C	1 min
1/2	62°C	2 min } (repeat 34 times)
1/3	72°C	3 min
2/1	72°C	7 min (repeat once)

9600 Thermocycler (Perkin-Elmer Cetus):

Cycle/step	Temperature	Time
1/1	94°C	10 s
1/2	62°C	1 min } (repeat 34 times)
1/3	72°C	2 min, 15 s
2/1	72°C	7 min (repeat once)

3.3. Gel Electrophoresis and Southern Analysis

Following the completion of PCR:

1. Remove 20 µL from each reaction, transferred to a new tube (if oil was used, be sure to wipe off the tip).
2. Add loading dye.
3. Run each sample on a 1.2% agarose TBE gel at 80 V with appropriate size markers.
4. Southern transfer the gel onto a nitrocellulose or nylon membrane (*see* Note 8).
5. Hybridize with the *NPM-ALK* junction specific probe, (2;5)-P, which has been end-labeled with ^{32}P using polynucleotide kinase.
6. Wash the blots at room temperature for 30 min in 2X SSC, 0.1% SDS, then for 30 min at 50°C also in 2X SSC, 0.1% SDS.
7. Autoradiograph and develop after 4 h of exposure (*see* Notes 9–12).

4. Notes

1. DMSO reduces secondary structure of the template that can interfere with extension by polymerase.
2. DTT is required for stabilization of some enzymes.
3. RNasin is an RNase inhibitor.
4. One key to successful RT-PCR is the quality of the starting RNA. Since RNA is easily degraded once it is in solution, RT-PCR is best performed on samples recently extracted.
5. Owing to degradation of RNA during tissue fixation and processing, it may be difficult to get good RNA from samples that have been formalin-fixed and paraffin-embedded *(19)*.

6. As with any PCR procedure, contamination is always possible. As mentioned before, single-run aliquots of reagents should be used along with dedicated pipetors. A separate set of pipetors should be used for nesting reactions.

7. Random hexamer primers (Pharmacia, Piscataway, NJ) may be used at a final concentration of 5 pmol/μL for the RT reaction instead of the (2;5)3'A and *NPM*3'A oligo primers, if desired, with good result.

8. Although the bands should be visible with ethidium bromide staining, it is important to do a Southern transfer of the gel onto a nitrocellulose or nylon membrane, then hybridize with the *NPM-ALK* junction specific probe in order to definitively establish the identity of the PCR products.

9. Signals should be of sufficient intensity to give a good autoradiograph following 4 h of exposure, although an overnight exposure is sometimes required.

10. If no signals are seen following PCR, the following steps should be taken:
    a. If no bands are present in the *NPM* controls, the RNA may not be clean enough to amplify. To clean, extract with phenol/chloroform/isoamyl alcohol, followed by extraction with chloroform/isoamyl alcohol, then precipitate the aqueous phase in NaOAc and ethanol.
    b. A second explanation for the lack of visible bands on an ethidium-stained gel is that one or more reagents are not good. RT and PCR reagents that are freeze-thawed multiple times (which shouldn't occur with single use aliquots), or that are stored in a freezer that doesn't keep constant temperature, may go bad.

11. If the bands seen are weak, or many additional bands are seen, it may be necessary to optimize the PCR conditions for your own use. Key factors for amplification by PCR appear to be: pH of the buffer; Mg^{2+}, dNTP, primer, and *Taq* polymerase concentrations; presence or absence of a cosolvent such as DMSO; and the cycling parameters.

12. If the bands on the gel look good, but there is no signal in Southern hybridizations, check the specific activities of the probes being used. A band of altered size may be seen in the occasional cases of t(2;5)-positive NHL that possess variant *NPM-ALK* fusion junctions (in our studies to date, one of 31 analyzed cases) *(4,7)*. The *NPM-ALK* product generated from these samples will not hybridize to oligo (2,5)-P, which is homologous to *NPM* and *ALK* sequences present at the usual fusion junction. Such variant fusions may be detectable in hybridizations using one of the two nesting oligos as probes, depending on the location of the fusion junctions in *NPM* and *ALK*.

Acknowledgments

Supported in part by National Institutes of Health, grants No. CA-01702 and CA-69129 (S. W. M.) and CA-01429 (J. R. D.), by Cancer Center Core grant No. CA-21765, by American Cancer Society (ACS) grant No. BE-218 (J. R. D.), and by the American Lebanese Syrian Associated Charities (ALSAC), St. Jude Children's Research Hospital.

References

1. Stein, H. and Dallenbach, F. (1992) Diffuse large cell lymphomas of B- and T-cell type, in *Neoplastic Hematopathology* (Knowles, D. M., ed.), Williams and Wilkins, Baltimore, pp. 675–714.
2. Lo Coco, F., Ye, B. H., Lista, F., Corradini, P., Offit, K., Knowles, D. M., Chaganti, R. S. K., and Dalla-Favera, R. (1994) Rearrangements of the BCL6 gene in diffuse large cell non-Hodgkin's lymphoma. *Blood* **83,** 1757–1759.
3. Bastard, C., Deweindt, C., Kerckaert, J. P., Lenorrnand, B., Rossi, A., Pezzella, F., Fruchart, C., Duval, C., Monconduit, M., and Tilly, H. (1994) *LAZ3* rearrangements in non-Hodgkin's lymphoma: correlation with histology, immunophenotype, karyotype, and clinical outcome in 217 patients. *Blood* **83,** 2423–2427.
4. Morris, S. W., Kirstein, M. N., Valentine, M. B., Dittmer, K. G., Shapiro, D. N., Saltman, D. L., and Look, A. T. (1994) Fusion of a kinase gene, *ALK*, to a nucleolar protein gene, *NPM*, in non-Hodgkin's lymphoma. *Science* **263,** 1281–1284.
5. Kadin, M. E. (1994) Ki-1/CD30+ (anaplastic) large-cell lymphoma: maturation of a clinicopathologic entity with prospects of effective therapy. *J. Clin. Oncol.* **12,** 884–887.
6. Greer, J. P., Kinney, M. C., Collins, R. D., Salhany, K. E., Wolff, S. N., Hainsworth, J. D., Flexner, J. M., and Stein, R. S. (1991) Clinical features of 31 patients with Ki-1 anaplastic large-cell lymphoma. *J. Clin. Oncol.* **9,** 539–547.
7. Downing, J. R., Shurtleff, S. A., Zielenska, M., Curcio-Brint, A. M., Behm, F. G., Head, D. R., Sandlund, J. T., Weisenburger, D. D., Kossakowska, A. E., Thorner, P., Lorenzano, A., Ladanyi, M., and Morris, S. W. (1995) Molecular detection of the t(2;5) translocation of non-Hodgkin's lymphoma by reverse transcriptase-polymerase chain reaction. *Blood* **85,** 3416–3422.
8. Borer, R. A., Lehner, C. F., Eppenberger, H. M., and Nigg, E. A. (1989) Major nucleolar proteins shuttle between nucleus and cytoplasm. *Cell* **56,** 379–390.
9. Chan, W. Y., Liu, Q. R., Boringin, J., Busch, H., Rennert, O., Tease, L., and Chan, P. K. (1989) Characterization of the cDNA encoding human nucleophosmin and studies of its role in normal and abnormal growth. *Biochemistry* **28,** 1033–1039.
10. Leoncini, L., Del Vecchio, M. T., Kra, R., Megha, T., Barbini, P., Cevenini, G., Poggi, S., Pileri, S., Tosi, P., and Cottier, H. (1990) Hodgkin's disease and CD30-positive anaplastic large cell lymphomas—a continuous spectrum of malignant disorders. A quantitative morphometric and immunohistologic study. *Am. J. Pathol.* **137,** 1047–1057.
11. Downing, J. R., Ladanyi, M., Raffeld, M., Weiss, L. M., and Morris, S. W. (1995) Large-cell anaplastic lymphoma-specific translocation in Hodgkin's disease (letter). *Lancet* **345,** 918,919.
12. Chan, W. C., Elmberger, G., Lozano, M. D., Sanger, W., and Weisenburger, D. D. (1995) Large-cell anaplastic lymphoma-specific translocation in Hodgkin's disease (letter). *Lancet* **345,** 921.
13. Orscheschek, K., Merz, H., Hell, J., Binder, T., Bartels, H., and Feller, A. C. (1995) Large-cell anaplastic lymphoma-specific translocation [t(2;5)(p23;q35)] in Hodgkin's disease: indication of a common pathogenesis. *Lancet* **345,** 87–89.

14. Ladanyi, M., Parsa, N. Z., Offit, K., Wachtel, M. S., Filippa, D. A., and Jhanwar, S. C. (1991) Clonal cytogenetic abnormalities in Hodgkin's disease. *Genes Chromosomes Cancer* **3**, 294–299.
15. Poppema, S., Kaleta, J., and Hepperle, B. (1992) Chromosomal abnormalities in patients with Hodgkin's disease: evidence for frequent involvement of the 14q chromosomal region but infrequent bcl-2 gene rearrangement in Reed-Sternberg cells. *J. Natl. Cancer Inst.* **84**, 1789–1793.
16. Chomczynski, P. and Sacchi, N. (1987) Single-step method of RNA isolation by acid guanidinium thiocyanate- phenol-chloroform extraction. *Anal. Biochem.* **162**, 156–159.
17. Dalton, W. T., Aheam, M. J., McCredie, K. B., Freireich, E. G., Stass, S. A., and Trujillo, J. M. (1988) HL60 cell line was derived from a patient with FAB-M2 and not FAB-M3. *Blood* **71**, 242–247.
18. Morgan, R., Smith, S. D., Hecht, B. K., Christy, V., Mellentin, J. D., Warnke, R., and Cleary, M. L. (1989) Lack of involvement of the c-ns and N-myc genes by chromosomal translocation t(2;5) (p23;q35) common to malignancies with features of so-called malignant histocytosis. *Blood* **73**, 2155–2164.
19. Lopategui, J. R., Sun, L.-H., Chan, J. K. C., Gaffey, M. J., Frieson, H. F., Glackin, C., and Weiss, L. M. (1995) Low frequency association of the t(2;5) (p23;q35) chromosomal translocation with CD30+ lymphomas from American and Asian patients: A reverse transcriptase-polymerase chain reaction study. *Am. J. Pathol.* **146**, 323–327.

8

Molecular Diagnosis of the 5q Deletion in Malignant Myeloid Disorders

Jackie Boultwood

1. Introduction

The 5q- chromosome is found in a spectrum of malignant myeloid disorders *(1)*. The 5q deletion is the most commonly reported deletion in the myelodysplastic syndromes (MDS) and is found in 10–15% of patients *(1)*. The 5q- chromosome occurs as a sole karyotypic abnormality in the distinct myelodysplastic syndrome the 5q- syndrome *(2)*. The 5q- chromosome is also observed frequently in therapy related MDS and acute myeloid leukemia (AML) where it is typically reported together with other karyotypic abnormalities *(3)*. The 5q deletion is interstitial and the breakpoints are variable. The breakpoints most frequently reported are 5q12-q14 (proximal) and 5q31-q33(distal) *(4)*. The most commonly reported 5q deletion is the del (5)(q13q33) *(5)*. There appears to be no difference in the pattern of 5q deletion breakpoints between MDS and AML *(4,5)*.

It has been postulated that the distal portion of the long arm of chromosome 5 contains a myeloid tumor suppressor gene and that this gene maps within the minimal deleted segment, termed the "critical region" of gene loss *(6)*. The proposed site of the critical region of gene loss of the 5q- chromosome varies between cytogenetic studies *(4,5)*. Recently, however, molecular and FISH techniques have been used by different groups to delineate the critical region(s) of the 5q- chromosome in precise molecular terms. These studies have resulted in the definition of more than one critical region predominantly mapping within 5q31. It is most probable that this reflects the different patient populations under investigation in these studies. The critical region of the 5q deletion in the 5q- syndrome has been defined by Boultwood et al. and maps to the approx 5 Mb region between the FGFA and NKSF1 genes (including CSF1R) *(7)*. Le Beau

From: *Methods in Molecular Medicine, Molecular Diagnosis of Cancer*
Edited by: F. E. Cotter Humana Press Inc., Totowa, NJ

et al. have defined the critical region of the 5q deletion in a range of malignant myeloid disorders as the approx 2.8 Mb region between the genes for IL9 and D5S166 (including EGR1) *(6)*. A more centromeric critical region mapping between the genes for IL5 and CSF2 and encompassing the IRF1 gene has been identified by Willman et al. in patients with MDS and AML *(8)*. Thus it is probable that there may be more than one myeloid tumor suppressor gene on 5q *(9)*. The delineation of more than one critical region of the 5q- chromosome is relevant to the approaches used for molecular diagnosis of this deletion. Although the majority of 5q deletions will be detected by the use of a single DNA marker mapping within 5q31 certain rare cases with either particularly small deletions or atypical deletion breakpoints may be missed. It is important, therefore, that in considering molecular diagnosis of the 5q- chromosome in malignant myeloid disorders due regard is given to the respective critical regions. The molecular techniques that commonly are employed for the identification of the 5q- deletion are essentially the same as those used for the detection of any chromosomal deletion in malignancy and all concern the detection of allelic loss. These techniques comprise restriction fragment length polymorphism (RFLP) analysis (either by Southern blotting or the polymerase chain reaction [PCR]), gene dosage studies and fluorescent "in situ" hybridization experiments (FISH). The practical details necessary to carry out these investigations in patients with malignant myeloid disorders are as follows.

2. Materials

2.1. Cell Separation

1. PBS/1 mM EDTA: 0.137M NaCl, 2.68 mM KCl, 7.98 mM Na$_2$HPO$_4$, 1.47 mM KH$_2$PO$_4$, pH 7.2, 1 mM EDTA.
2. Lysis buffer: 10 mM NaHCO$_3$, 0.15M NH$_4$Cl, 0.1 mM EDTA. The solution should be freshly prepared when required and filter sterilized before use.
3. Ficoll (Sigma, St. Louis, MO).
4. Histopaque (Sigma).
5. 22% bovine serum albumin.
6. 2% Alsevers (TCS Biologicals Ltd., Buckingham, UK): Neuraminidase treated sheep red blood cells.
7. Fetal calf serum (Sigma).
8. Polybrene (Sigma).

2.2. Southern Analysis

1. Hybond N (Amersham, Arlington Heights, IL).
2. Random hexanucleotides (Boehring Mannheim, Mannheim, Germany).
3. 20X Standard saline citrate (SSC-stock solution): 175.3 g of NaCl, 88.2 g of sodium citrate, 10N NaOH to adjust the pH to 7.0 and made up to 1 L with distilled water. Autoclave to sterilize.

4. 10% Sodium dodecylsulfate (SDS).
5. 50X Tris-acetate electrophoresis buffer (TAE-stock solution): 242 g Tris base, 57.1 mL glacial acetic acid, 100 mL of $0.5M$ EDTA (pH 8.0) made up to 1 L. Autoclave to sterilize.

2.3. RFLP Analysis by PCR

1. 10X PCR buffer; 500 mM KCl, 10 mM Tris-HCl, pH 8.3.
2. Deoxynucleotide triphosphates: 10 mM each of dATP, dCTP, dGTP, and, dTTP.
3. 25 mM MgCl$_2$.
4. Paraffin oil (Sigma).
5. *Taq* polymerase.

2.4. Microsatellite Polymorphism Analysis

1. Loading dye: 0.25% bromophenol blue, 0.25% xylene cyanol FF, and 15% Ficoll (Type 400) in dH$_2$O.
2. 10X Tris-borate electrophoresis buffer (TBE): 108 g Tris base, 55 g boric acid, 40 mL of 05M EDTA (ph 8.0), made up to 1 L. Autoclave to sterilize.

3. Methods

3.1. RFLP Analysis

RFLP analysis is used widely in the study of chromosomal loss in malignancy. Each gene has two (or more) alleles and these may be found in different forms, i.e., be polymorphic. RFLP analysis is dependent on these differences. When a given restriction enzyme site is present in the DNA sequence of one allele of a gene but absent from the second allele on the other homologous chromosome a correspondingly shorter DNA fragment will be produced from the former allele and a longer DNA fragment from the latter allele. Thus the two chromosomes may be distinguished on the basis of this RFLP in a heterozygous (or informative) individual. First, it is necessary to establish whether any given patient is informative for a particular RFLP. Subsequently, tumor DNA and control DNA (from an uninvolved tissue) is analyzed using a probe that detects a specific polymorphism. The control DNA would be expected to show fragments representing both alleles and the tumor DNA only one allele, the second allele having been lost as a result of the deletion. RFLP analysis by Southern blotting methodology and PCR is described.

3.1.1. Peripheral Blood Cell Fractionation

3.1.1.1. FICOLL SEPARATION

RFLP analysis is performed routinely on DNA samples from patient bone marrow or whole peripheral blood samples. However, it is preferable to carryout RFLP analysis on as pure a tumor cell population as may be obtained.

Peripheral blood cell fractionation using Ficoll centrifugation is used widely to prepare pure granulocyte (malignant sample), and mononuclear cell (control sample) fractions in patients with MDS (*see* Note 1). The mononuclear fraction may be further purified to pure T-lymphocytes by E-rosetting *(11)*. The separation of peripheral blood into fractions should be attempted for AML patients. These patients have a high proportion of blasts in the peripheral blood that are found predominantly in the mononuclear fraction.

3.1.1.2. Separation of Granulocytes and Mononuclear Cells

 1. Take 50 mL of peripheral blood into a sterile tube containing EDTA.
 2. Allow Histopaque (Sigma) to reach room temperature and pipet 25 mL into a conical centrifuge tube.
 3. Layer 25 mL of blood gently onto the Histopaque using a widebore pipet and centrifuge at 400*g* for 30 min at room temperature.
 4. Remove the upper layer to within 0.5 cm of the opaque interface carefully with a pipet. Transfer the opaque interface (mononuclear cell fraction) into a sterile centrifuge tube. Retain the tube containing the red cell layer (granulocyte fraction) for further processing (steps 9–17).
 5. Add 50 mL of PBS/1 m*M* EDTA to the mononuclear fraction and mix by gentle aspiration.
 6. Centrifuge at 400*g* for 10 min at room temperature. Pour off the supernatant and repeat washing step 5.
 7. Resuspend the cell pellet in 10 mL of PBS/1 m*M* EDTA and determine the cell concentration using an automated counter or a hemocytometer.
 8. Determine the purity of the cell population by preparing a cytospin slide. The cell concentration required for cytospin preparations is 1×10^6/mL. Mix two drops of cell suspension with one drop of 22% bovine albumin per slide and spin for 10 min in an appropriate cytospin.
 9. Remove the histopaque layer to within 0.5 cm of the red cell layer.
10. Add 50 mL of PBS/1 m*M* EDTA to the red cell layer and mix by gentle aspiration.
11. Centrifuge at 400*g* for 10 min at room temperature. Pipet off the supernatant and repeat step 10.
12. Distribute the packed red blood cells into centrifuge tubes containing lysis buffer (approx 1 mL of red blood cells to 50 mL of red cell lysis buffer). Mix by gentle inversion and leave at room temperature for 20 min.
13. Centrifuge at 400*g* for 10 min at room temperature and pour off the supernatant.
14. Resuspend the granuloyte fraction in 1 mL PBS/1 m*M* EDTA, pool into two centrifuge tubes.
15. Add PBS/1 m*M* EDTA to 50 mL. Centrifuge at 400*g* for 10 min at room temperature. Pour off the supernatant and repeat this washing procedure two further times.
16. Resuspend the cell pellet in 10 mL PBS/1 m*M* EDTA and determine the cell concentration using an automated counter or a hemocytometer.
17. Prepare cytospin slides to determine cell purity.

3.1.1.3. T-Cell Separation

1. Adjust the mononuclear cell concentration 2–6 × 10^6 cells/mL.
2. Add 0.5–1 vol of fetal calf serum, 1–2 vol of 2% sheep Alsevers (neuraminidase-treated sheep red blood cells) solution, and 5 mL 5% (in distilled water) stock solution of Polybrene.
3. Mix and centrifuge at 70g for 5 min at 4°C. Leave overnight (or a minimum of 5 h) at 4°C.
4. Remove the supernatant and resuspend the cells by gentle rotation of the tube at an angle where the meniscus passes through the cell pellet. Gently underlayer with an equal volume (approx 10 mL) of Histopaque (Sigma). Centrifuge at 400g for 30 min at room temperature.
5. Remove the upper interface by pipeting (B-lymphocytes and monocytes).
6. Resuspend (B-lymphocytes and monocytes) in 50 mL PBS/1 mM EDTA and centrifuge at 400g for 10 min at room temperature. Remove the supernatant and repeat washing step (only carry out this step if non-T-cells are required).
7. Pipet off the supernatant to the red cell layer and follow procedure for Ficoll separation of peripheral blood, steps 10–17, to prepare pure T-cells.

3.1.2. Southern Analysis

1. Prepare high-mol-wt DNA samples (*see* Chapter 6) from patient bone marrow samples, peripheral blood samples, or granulocyte and T-lymphocyte cell fractions (*see* Section 3.1.1.3.) as well as from the whole peripheral blood of 10 or more healthy controls.
2. Digest the DNA with an appropriate restriction enzyme and size fractionate by electrophoresis, through 1% (this may vary depending on the separation required) agarose gels (*see* Note 2).
3. Transfer the DNA to Hybond N (Amersham) according to standard procedures for Southern blotting (*see* Chapter 3).
4. Label the DNA probes to high specific activity by random hexanucleotide priming (Boehringer Mannheim) and hybridize the probes to the filters at 65°C for 16 h.
5. Wash the filters for 30 min in 0.1X standard saline citrate (SSC) containing 0.1% sodium dodecylsulfate (SDS) at 65°C.
6. Carry out autoradiography using X-ray film for 1–7 d at –70°C (*see* Note 3).

3.1.3. RFLP Detection by PCR

PCR is an in vitro method of nucleic acid synthesis by which a particular sequence of DNA can be replicated specifically. PCR may be used for RFLP analysis in malignancy. This methodology is particularly valuable in cases where patient material is limited because only very small amounts (ngs or less) of DNA are required for analysis. The preparation of very pure tumor samples (ideally, >95%) is important in this form of analysis. Incorrect or inconclusive results may be obtained if the proportion of contaminating normal tissue is high.

1. Prepare DNA samples (*see* Chapter 6) from MDS patient granulocyte and T-lymphocyte fractions (*see* Sections 3.1.1.2. and 3.1.1.3.) or mononuclear samples of AML patients as well as from the mononuclear of 10 healthy controls.
2. Obtain appropriate primer pairs flanking a known RFLP within a DNA sequence (*see* Note 4).
3. Carry out PCR reaction in 0.5 m*M* sterile microcentrifuge tube. The basic procedure for PCR amplification is as follows:

	Amount for 1 PCR	Final concentration
Sterile H_2O	72.5 µL	
10X PCR buffer	10 µL	1X
dNTPs	8 µL	200 µ*M* each
$MgCl_2$ (*see* Note 5)	6 µL	1.5 µ*M*
Oligonucleotide primer (forward)	1 µL	1 µ*M*
Oligonucleotide primer (reverse)	1 µL	1 µ*M*
Ampli *Taq* polymerase	0.5 µL	2.5 U
Final volume	99 µL	

4. Add 1 µL (1 µg) of the appropriate DNA template to the PCR reaction mix and mix gently by pipeting. Add 100 µL paraffin oil (Sigma).
5. Place the tubes on a DNA thermal cycler and perform amplification. The cycling profile will vary depending on the individual PCR experiments (*see* Note 6).
6. Digest the PCR products with an appropriate enzyme (i.e., that which cuts at a known polymorphic site) and electrophorese through an agarose gel (containing 0.4 µg/mL ethidium bromide) using a minigel system. The agarose concentration of the gel will vary from 1.5–4% depending on the size of the PCR product.
7. Visualize the products using a transilluminator. Allelic deletion is demonstrated when the tumor DNA shows loss of either the single uncut band or of the cut bands.

3.1.4. Nondenaturing Polyacrylamide Gel Electrophoresis for Detection of Microsatellite Polymorphisms

Interspersed repetitive DNA sequences in the form of dinucleotide repeats (especially [CA] and [GA]), trinucleotide repeats, and tetronucleotide repeats have been found to exhibit length polymorphisms. These are termed microsatellite polymorphisms and represent a valuable source of informative genetic markers. This type of polymorphism can be studied once the sequence encompassing the microsatellite has been determined. PCR primers unique to the region flanking the repeats is used to amplify the region of DNA obtained from a group of individuals. The analyzed fragments are then sized on nondenaturing polyacrylamide gels.

1. Obtain PCR primers specific for the region flanking the repeats (*see* Table 1).
2. Prepare DNA samples obtained from MDS patient granulocyte and T-lymphocyte blood fractions (*see* Sections 3.1.1.2. and 3.1.1.3.) or mononuclear samples of AML patients as well as from the mononuclear samples of 10 healthy controls.

Table 1
Chromosome 5 Microsatellite Polymorphisms Mapping 5q23–33

Locus	Heterozygosity rate	Cytogenetic position	Linkage map position
IL9	0.62	q22.3-q31.3	D5S58-D5S52
D5S210	0.75	q22-q22.3 or q31.3-q33.3	D5S54-D5S55
D5S207	0.69	q22-q22.3 or q31.3-q33.3	D5S52-D5S55
CSF1R	0.86	q22-q22.3 or q31.3-q33.3	D5S52-D5S61
D5S209	0.71	q22-q22.3 or q31.3-q33.3	D5S54-D5S61
D5S119	0.49	q22-q22.3 or q33.1-q33.3	D5S52-D5S43

3. Perform PCR amplification on patient and control DNA (*see* Section 3.1.3.).
4. Prepare a 6 or 10% polyacrylamide gel in 1X TBE.
5. Mount gel on suitable Electrophoresis apparatus, e.g., protein II electrophoresis Apparatus (Bio-Rad, Richmond, CA).
6. Mix 6–30 µL of PCR products with a tenth volume of loading dye.
7. Load the samples on the polyacrylamide gel and electrophorese in 1X TBE at 300 V for 4–5 h at 18°C.
8. Stain the gel with ethidium bromide (0.4 µg/mL) and visualize the bands on a transilluminator.

3.2. Gene Dosage Analysis

The value of RFLP analysis to the detection of chromosomal deletion is entirely dependent upon the informative rate (heterozygosity) of the probe of interest. If this is low then the loss status of only a small proportion of the patients under investigation will be determinable. Gene dosage analysis, however, will allow for an assessment of the allelic loss on every patient with any probe *(7,8)*.

In addition this methodology allows for a quantitative assessment of gene loss (loss of one or both alleles). Gene dosage is not, however, as sensitive as RFLP analysis and is only reliable if carefully controlled. In these experiments nylon filters containing patient DNA samples and control DNA samples are simultaneously hybridized with two probes, a probe for the gene of interest and a probe for a gene present on a chromosome known to be uninvolved in the particular patient population (i.e., karyotypically normal) that acts as an internal hybridization standard. After autoradiography the film is scanned with a densitometer to quantitative the relative intensities of the two hybridization signals (*see* Fig. 1A and B).

1. Prepare DNA samples (*see* Chapter 6) obtained from MDS patient granulocyte and T-lymphocyte blood fractions (*see* Sections 3.1.1.2. and 3.1.1.3.) and mononuclear samples of AML patients as well as from the mononuclear samples of 10 healthy controls.

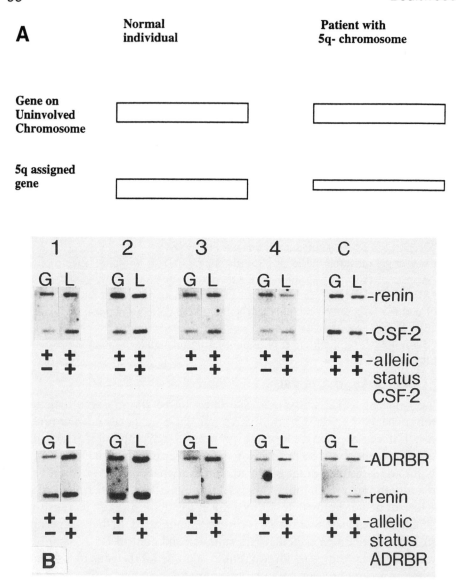

Fig. 1. (A) Schematic illustration of gene dosage analysis. **(B)** Loss of CSF2 and ADRB2 in patients with a 5q deletion. DNA samples from the lymphocyte fraction (lane L) and granulocyte fraction (lane G) from patients (numbers 1–4) and from a healthy normal control (C) were digested with *Eco*R1 and hybridized simultaneously to the genomic renin probe and either the genomic CSF2 probe or the ADRB2 probe. Optical densitometric readings were used to obtain comparative ratios between the two signals. The presence of two alleles is designated as ++ and loss of one of two alleles as +–. Numbers 1–4 show deletion of one CSF2 allele and one ADRB2 allele from the granulocyte fraction (+–). The lymphocyte fraction of numbers 1–4 as well as the granulocyte and lymphocyte fraction from the normal control show no loss of either CSF2 or ADRB2 (++).

Table 2
Gene Dosage Analysis in 5q31

Chromosome 5 gene of interest	Recommended probe mix	Reference
1RF1	1RF1 cDNA fragment—clone HHC PS21 and 1.9 kb genomic *Eco*RI-*Sst*I fragment of renin gene	*18*
EGR1	EGR1 primer pair generated probe of 337 bp CCACCTCTTAGGTCAGATGGAAG TCCATGGCACAGATGCTGTAC (annealing temperature 57°C) and 1.9 kb genomic *Eco*RI-*Sst*I fragment of renin gene	*7*
CSF1R	3 kb genomic *Eco*R1 fragment of CSF1R gene (5') and 1.9 kb genomic *Eco*R1-*Sst*I fragment of renin gene	*19*

2. Digest the DNA samples with an appropriate restriction enzyme and carry out gel electrophoresis and Southern blotting as described previously (*see* Note 7).
3. The resulting filters should be simultaneously hybridized with two probes; a probe for the gene of interest on chromosome 5 and a probe for a second gene present on a different chromosome (known to be karyotypically normal in the series of patients under investigation) that acts as an internal hybridization standard (*see* Table 2 for precise details of probe combinations appropriate for diagnosis of the 5q- chromosome in different myeloid disorders).
4. Following washing and autoradiography, scan the film using an enhanced lazer densitometer (LKB Ultrascan XL, Bromma, Sweden) to quantitate the relative intensities of the two hybridization signals.
5. Derive a comparative densitometric ratio from the two hybridization signals in 10 normal individuals. An approx 50% reduction in this ratio indicates a 50% reduction in the dosage of the chromosome 5 assigned gene of interest and is consistent with the loss of one allele.
6. Repeat the gene dosage experiments two further times.

3.3. FISH Analysis

FISH analysis (*see* Chapter 13) allows for the localization of DNA probes ranging from 1 kb to whole YACs (100–1000 kb) on metaphase chromosomes. This technique makes possible the rapid mapping of such DNA probes with >1 Mb resolution. Fish techniques are now being widely used for the detection of chromosomal deletions in tumor cells[6]. Cosmids or YACS mapping to the critical regions of the 5q- chromosome may be used to identify this karyotypic abnormality in malignant myeloid disorders. The methodology necessary for FISH analysis is detailed in Chapter 13. It is recommended that the investigation employs DNA markers mapping within each of the three critical region mapping to 5q31 in order to be confident of 100% detection of 5q- chromosomes in these disorders. Cosmids or YACs encompassing IRF1, EGR1, and CSF1R are ideal for such studies.

4. Notes

1. The nature of the progenitor cell affected in MDS and AML has been the subject of several studies with some indicating that a common myeloid-lymphoid stem cell is involved in the disorder, whereas others have proposed that the disease originates in a progenitor cell committed to the myeloid lineage. Overall the literature would suggest that in the majority of patients with MDS the granulocyte fraction is monoclonal (affected) and the T-lymphocyte fractions polyclonal (unaffected). In patients with the 5q- syndrome two reports suggest that myeloid but not lymphoid cells harbor the 5q- chromosome.

2. The enzyme of choice will be that for which a group of individuals are polymorphic at a given DNA sequence. Suitable RFLPs for the detection of the 5q- chromosome in different malignant myeloid disorders are shown in Table 3 and Fig 2.

3. The film may be scanned using an enhanced lazer densitometer (LKB, Ultrascan XL) to quantitate the relative intensities of the hybridization signals from the allelic fragments in normal individuals as compared to tumor samples. However, if pure tumor samples have been studied the reduction in the intensity of one allelic fragment (mapping within the deleted region) to the other (present on the homologous karyotypically normal chromosome) will be very marked and analysis by eye should suffice.

4. The APC and MCC genes have been localized to 5q22 and a large number of PCR-based polymorphism analyses with high heterozygosity rates have been identified for these genes. Although these genes map outside of the critical region of the 5q- chromosome at 5q31 the majority of patients with the 5q- deletion will have loss of this region. Recommended polymorphisms include the SspI polymorphism in the sequence encoding the 3' untranslated region of the APC gene *(16)*.

	Digest products	Frequency
a1	270, 580 bp	0.46
a2	135, 135, 580 bp	0.54

5. The $MgCl_2$ concentration may vary depending on the primer and template used. Optimization of the PCR may be performed by using concentrations of $MgCl_2$ between 1.5 and 4.0 µM

6. PCR cycling temperatures normally used are as follows: denaturation of the DNA strands at 94°C, annealing of primers to templates 50–65°C, extension of primers at 72°C. The period of time to which PCR reactions are exposed to these tem-

Table 3
Polymorphic Human DNA Segments Mapping to Distal Portion of 5q

Map location	Locus symbol	Probe	Enzyme	Constant bands	Allele		Reference
					Symbol size	Frequency (kb)	
5q23-31	IL3	gIL-cDNA	*Bgl*II	—	A1 19.1	0.90	*13*
					A2 15.4	0.10	
5q31	DS589	2 kb *HindIII* fragment of DS589	*EcoRI*	—	C1 5.3		*14*
				—	C2 3.5		
5q31q33	CSF1R	3.8 kb *EcoRI* cDNA	*EcoRI*	3.0, 2.5	A1 29	0.14	*15*
					A2 16, 13	0.86	

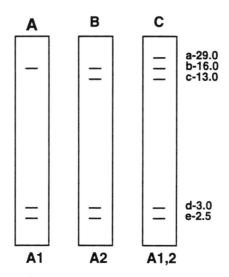

Fig. 2. RFLP analysis at the CSF1R locus. (*See* Table 1 for details.)

peratures is 1–3 min. The number of cycles performed varies from 15–40 cycles. All PCR reactions are subjected to an initial denaturation step of 94°C for 8 min to ensure that the template DNA is completely denatured.

7. Preliminary experiments should be carried out in order to determine the restriction enzyme that is most appropriate for any given gene dosage study, i.e., ideally that which results in single hybridization fragments for each of the two genes under investigation.

References

1. Van den Berghe, H., Vermaelen, K., Mecucci, C., Barbieri, D., and Tricot, G. (1985) The 5q- anomaly. *Cancer Genet. Cytogenet.* **17**, 189–255.
2. Van den Berghe, H., Cassiman, J. J, David, G., Fryns, J. P., Michaux, J. L, and Sokal, G. (1974) Distinct haematological disorder with deletion of the long arm of No. 5 chromosome. *Nature* **251**, 437–438.
3. Le Beau, M. M., Albain, K. S., Larson, R. A., Vardiman, J. W., Davis, E. M., Blough, R. R., Golomb, H. M., and Rowley, J. D. (1986) Clinical and cytogenetic correlations in 63 patients with therapy-related myelodysplastic syndromes and acute non-lymphocytic leukemia: further evidence for characteristic abnormalities of chromosomes nos 5 and 7. *J. Clin. Oncol.* **4**, 325–345.
4. Mitelman, F., Manolova, Y., Manolova, G., Billstom, R., Heims, S., Kristofferson, U., and Mandahl, N. (1986) Analysis of the 5q marker chromosome in refractory anemia. *Hereditas* **105**, 49–54.
5. Pedersen, B. and Jensen, I. M. (1991) Clinical and prognostic implications of chromosome 5q deletions: 96 high resolution studied patients. *Leukemia* **5**, 566–573.

6. Le Beau, M. M., Espinosa, R., Neuman, W. L., Stock, W., Roulston, D., Larson, R. A., Keinanen, M., and Westbrook, C. A. (1993) Cytogenetic and molecular delieation of the smallest commonly deleted region of chromosome 5 in malignant myeloid diseases. *Proc. Natl. Acad. Sci. USA* **90**, 5484–5488.
7. Boultwood, J., Fidler, C., Lewis, S., Kelly, S., Sheridan, H., Littlewood, T. J., Buckle, V. J., and Wainscoat, J. S. (1994) Molecular Mapping of uncharacteristically small 5q deletions in two patients with the 5q- syndrome: delineation of the critical region on 5q and identification of a 5q- breakpoint. *Genomics* **19**, 425–432.
8. Willman, C. .L, Sever, C. E., Pallavicini, M. G., Harada, H., Tanaka, N., Slovak, M.L., Yamamoto, H., Harada, K., Meeker, T. C., List, A. F., et al (1993) Deletion of IRF-1, mapping to chromosome 5q31.1, in human leukemia and preleukemic myelodysplasia. *Science* **259**, 968–71.
9. Boultwood, J., Lewis, S., and Wainscoat, J. S. (1994) The 5q- syndrome. *Blood* **84**, 3253.
10. Boyum, A. (1986) Isolation of mononuclear cells and granulocytes from human blood: isolation of mononuclear cells by one centrifugation and of granulocytes by combining centrifugation and sedimentation at 1g. *Scand. J. Clin. Lab. Invest.* **97**, 77(suppl).
11. Kaplan, M. E. and Clark, C. J. (1974) An improved rosetting assay for detection of human T-lymphocytes. *J. Immunol. Methods* **5**, 131.
12. Mullis, K. B. and Faloona, F. A. (1987) Specific synthesis of DNA in vitro via a polymerase-catalyzed chain reaction. *Methods Enzymol.* **155**, 335–350.
13. Weber, J. L. and May, P. E. (1989) Abundant class of human DNA polymorphisms which can be typed using the polymerase chain reaction. *Am. J. Hum. Genet.* **81**, 388–396.
14. Nagarajan, L., Zavadil, J., Claxton, D., Lu, X., Fairman, J., Warrington, J., Wasmuth, J. J., Chinault, A. C., Sever, C. E., Slovak, M. L., Willman, C. L., and Deisseroth, A. B. (1994) Consistent Loss of the D5S89 locus mapping telomeric to the interleukin gene cluster and centromeric to EGR-1 in patients with 5q- chromosome. *Blood* **83**, 199–208.
15. De Qi, Xu, Guilhot, S., and Galibert, F. (1985) Restriction fragment length polymorphism of the human c-fms gene. *PNAS* **82**, 2862–2865.
16. Heighway, J., Hoban, P. R., and Wyllie, A. H. (1991) Sspl polymorphism in sequence encoding 3' untranslated region of the APC gene. *Nucl. Acids Res.* **19**, 6966.
17. Weber, J. L., Polymeropoulos, M. H., May, P. E., Kwitek, A. E., Xiao, H., McPherson, J. D., and Wasmuth, J. J. (1991) *Genomics* **11**, 695–700.
18. Boultwood, J., Fidler, C., Lewis, S., MacCarthy, A., Sheridan, H., Littlewood, T. J., Buckle, V. J., and Wainscoat, J. S. (1993) Allelic loss of IRF1 in myelodysplasia and acute myeloid leukemia: Retention of IRF1 on the 5q- chromosome in some patients with the 5q- syndrome. *Blood* 2611–2616.
19. Boultwood, J., Rack, K., Kelly, S., Madden, J., Sakoguchi, A. Y., Wang, L. M., Oscier, D. G., Buckle, V. J., and Wainscoat, J. S. (1991) Loss of both FMS alleles in patients with myelodysplasia and a chromosome 5 deletion. *Proc. Natl. Acad. Sci. USA 88,* 6176.

9

Polymerase Chain Reaction Based Methods for Assessing Chimerism Following Allogeneic Bone Marrow Transplantation

Mark Lawler and Shaun R. McCann

1. Introduction

It is important to be able to assess the contribution of donor cells to the graft following bone marrow transplantation (BMT), as complete engraftment of marrow progenitors that can give rise to long term donor derived hemopoiesis may be important in long-term disease-free survival. The contribution of the donor marrow, both in terms of filling the marrow "space" created by the intense conditioning regimen and in its ability to mediate a graft versus leukemia effect may be assessed by studying the kinetics of the engraftment process. As BMT involves repopulation of the host hemopoietic system with donor cells, recipients of allogeneic marrow are referred to as hemopoietic chimeras. A donor chimera is an individual who exhibits complete donor hemopoiesis and we would imagine that donor chimerism carries the best long-term prognosis. A patient who has both donor and recipient cells coexisting in a stable fashion post-BMT without hematological evidence of relapse or graft rejection is referred to as a mixed chimera. Mixed chimerism may be a prelude to graft rejection or leukemic relapse; therefore, it is important to be able to monitor the presence of these cells in a precise manner.

A variety of methods are used to assess chimerism post-BMT. As these methods vary in their detection sensitivities and in the types of cell they examine, the reported incidence of mixed chimerism may vary. Karyotypic analysis has been applied widely in this area but is at its most useful in sex mismatched transplants where the Y chromosome can be used as a marker of engraftment. Protein polymorphisms are generally applicable to a single cell type and thus may misrepresent the contribution of donor cells to multi-lineage engraftment,

From: *Methods in Molecular Medicine, Molecular Diagnosis of Cancer*
Edited by: F. E. Cotter Humana Press Inc., Totowa, NJ

particularly when studying situations such as the immunotherapeutic effect of donor leukocyte infusions. Both karyotyping and protein polymorphisms suffer from low sensitivity in detection of the minor cell population. While sensitivity can be increased by erythrocyte antigen typing, results in the early post-BMT period may be complicated by blood or platelet transfusions.

DNA methodologies, either by the use of restriction fragment length polymorphisms (RFLPs) and variable number tandem repeats (VNTRs) combined with Southern blotting, or more recently by using the polymerase chain reaction (PCR), allow all nucleated cell types to be examined in a single sample. These markers rely on the polymorphic nature of human genome; variation in either restriction enzyme sites or in the number of tandem repeats between donor and recipient provides a sensitive and straightforward marker of engraftment *(1,2)*. The increased sensitivity of the PCR-based methods permits sensitive detection of minor cell populations. Initial PCR assays involved the use of primers for DNA sequences specific to the Y chromosome *(3,4)*. Use of Y-specific PCR is ideally suited to situations where the recipient is male and the donor is female as reemerging recipient cells can be correlated with the appearance of a Y-specific signal. PCR of VNTRs, however, does not limit studies to sex mismatched situations and has proved to be extremely reliable and is now widely used in the detection of minor cell populations *(5)*. The discovery of a new form of genetic variation called microsatellites and short tandem repeats (STRs), which also show variation in the number of a repeat motif between individuals *(6)*, has also proved to be a very useful method in the assessment of chimerism *(7)*.

Microsatellites have a repeat length of 2 bp of the form the Cytosine Adenine dinucleotide(dC; dA; dG; dT) whereas in STRs the repeat unit can range from 2 to 5 bp and have a variety of different core repeat sequence motifs (e.g. TTTA CAG). This review will focus on the use of PCR-based methods for assessing chimerism due to their high sensitivity and robust nature. Southern blot based methods will only be referred to briefly; readers are referred to a variety of references for more detail of these methods *(1,2)*.

2. Solutions and Materials

2.1. DNA Extraction from Peripheral Blood and Bone Marrow

1. RPMI medium.
2. Lymphoprep (Ficoll).
3. 10% Sodium dodecy sulfate (SDS).
4. Proteinase K (10 mg/mL).
5. Tris-saturated phenol (1:1 ratio of phenol and 0.5*M* Tris-HCl, pH 7.5).
6. 8 hydroxyquinoline (0.1 g/100 mL).
7. Phenol chloroform (1/1).
8. 3*M* Sodium acetate (Na Ac).
9. Ethanol.

2.2. Extraction of DNA from Stored Hematological Slides
1. Noindet P40(0.1%).
2. Lysis buffer: 10 m*M* Tris-HCl, pH 7.8, 10 m*M* NaCl, 10 m*M* EDTA, 1% SDS, and 2 μg/mL proteinase K.
3. Xylene.

2.3. Buccal Wash DNA Preparation
1. 15% saline.
2. 1% SDS.
3. 10 mg/mL proteinase K.

2.4. PCR of Y Chromosome Specific Sequences
1. Ammonium hydroxide (NH_4OH) 10% solution.
2. Phenol/chloroform (1/1).
3. PCR buffer: 50 m*M* KCl, 10 m*M* Tris-HCl, pH 8.3, 1.5 m*M* $MgCl_2$, and 0.01% gelatin (*see* Note 1).

2.5. PCR of Variable Number Tandem Repeat Sequences (VNTR-PCR)
1. Sample loading buffer: 100 m*M* TBE, 2 mm EDTA, 0.5% bromophenol blue, 0.5% xylene cyanol, 30% Ficoll Hypaque.
2. Polynucleotide kinase (10 U/μL).
3. Kinase buffer: 10X 500 m*M* Tris-HCl, pH 7.5, 100 m*M* $MgCl_2$, 50 m*M* DTT, 1 m*M* spermidine.
4. $\gamma^{32}P$ dATP (3000 Ci/mmol, Amersham, UK).
5. Washing solution: 1X SSC, 1% SDS.
6. X-ray film (Kodak, Rochester, NY;AGFA, Belgium).

2.6. Short Tandem Repeat PCR (STR-PCR)
1. PCR buffer: 50 m*M* KCl, 10 m*M* Tris-HCl, pH 8.3, 1.5 m*M* $MgCl_2$, and 0.01% gelatin.
2. "Hot" dNTP: Mix 2 m*M* dGTP, 2 m*M* dATP, 2 m*M* dTTP.
3. *Taq* polymerase (Perkin Elmer, Cheshire, UK; Emeryville, CA).
4. 10X Tris-borate electrophoresis buffer (TBE) (108 g Tris-base, 55 g boric acid, 40 mL 0.5*M* EDTA [pH 8.0]). Adjust volume up to 1 L with double-distilled water (ddH_2O).
5. 20% Polyacrylamide bis-acrylamide stock: 193 g acrylamide (DNA sequencing grade), 6.7 g *N,N*'-methylenebisacrylamide, 100 mL 10X TBE. Add 600 mL of ddH_2O and mix on a heated stirrer. Adjust volume to 1 L with ddH_2O. Filter solution and store in glass bottles surrounded with tinfoil at room temperature. All weighing of compounds should be done in a fume hood as acrylamide is a potent neurotoxin.
6. 7.75*M* Urea: 233.5 g urea, 50 mL 10X TBE. Adjust volume to 500 mL with ddH_2O.
7. 10% Ammonium persulfate: Make up 6 mL in 600-μL aliquots, which may be stored at –20°C for 1–2 wk.
8. $\alpha^{32}P$ dCTP.
9. 25–100 μ*M* dCTP.

3. Methods

There are a variety of sources of material routinely available for chimerism studies post-BMT. Bone-marrow aspirates, peripheral blood samples and stored hematological slides can be used to analyze the contribution of donor and recipient to multilineage engraftment. In addition, the chimeric status of various lineages may be studied using a variety of cell separation and purification techniques *(8–11)*. PCR also allows analysis of crude lysates or even directly of blood without prior purification *(12)*.

Chimerism studies using Southern-based methodologies require high-mol-wt DNA. This can be isolated from a 20-mL blood sample using a variety of techniques. Triton solubilization of centrifuged nuclei *(13)* followed by digestion overnight with proteinase K/SDS yields high quality DNA after phenol/chloroform extraction and ethanol precipitation *(see ref. 14)* Alternatively heparinized blood can be initially layered on Ficoll Hypaque to select mononuclear cells for analysis.

3.1. DNA Extraction from Peripheral Blood (PB) or Bone Marrow Aspirates (BM) (see Note 2)

1. Mix 3 mL PB with 10 mL RPMI medium and layer onto Lymphoprep. (If adding BM, there is no need to dilute with RPMI unless marrow is hypercellular.)
2. Spin at 1800 rpm (2215g) for 25 min. Remove buffy coat and centrifuge for 10 min at 2215g. Wash pellet in RPMI/MEM medium.
3. Lyse cells by adding 1/100 vol of the SDS solution followed by 1/10 vol of the proteinase K solution.
4. Allow cells to lyse overnight at 37°C.
5. Extract with phenol with 8 hydroxyquinoline added to the phenol to prevent oxidation. (This mixture can be stored at 4°C in the dark for several weeks.) Remove aqueous layer and repeat procedure.
6. Perform a final extraction with phenol chloroform, making sure to remove only the aqueous layer.
7. Add 1/10 vol 3*M* NaAc and 2 vol ice-cold ethanol. Place at −70° for 30 min and extract DNA either by spooling (for large amounts of DNA) or by centrifugation.
8. Perform one or two 70% ethanol washes and resuspend in ddH₂O. Leave at room temperature for 24 h to allow DNA to dissolve fully and aliquot into stock and working aliquots.

3.2. Extraction of DNA from Stored Hematological Slides

1. Scrape off material into a 1.5-mL Eppendorf tube using a sterile scalpel blade (*see* Notes 3–5).
2. Centrifuge for 5 s to bring all powdered material to the bottom of the Eppendorf.
3. Resuspend pelleted cells in 500 μL of a Nonidet solution for 15 min to lyse cells.
4. Centrifuge and incubate the nuclear pellets in 150–200 μL of lysis buffer.
5. Incubate overnight at 37°C.

6. Phenol and chloroform extract.
7. Ethanol precipitate as already described.

3.3. Buccal Wash DNA Prep (see Note 6)

1. Sluice oral cavity with 10 mL of a saline solution.
2. Collect material in a 15-mL tube and centrifuge at 10,000 rpm (12,310g) to pellet cells.
3. Resuspend pellet in 300 μL ddH$_2$O and add 3 μL 1% SDS and 30 μL proteinase K.
4. Incubate overnight at 37°C and extract as previously described.

Having established the methods available to access DNA from either fresh or archival hematological material, we will now examine the methods available for PCR-based DNA analysis.

3.4. PCR of Y Chromosome Specific Sequences (see Note 7)

One of the earliest PCR-based systems involved the use of Y-specific primers in the assessment of chimerism following sex mismatched transplants. Primers can be designed to a variety of Y-specific sequences (Fig. 1, Table 1).

1. Primers are synthesized on a DNA synthesizer such as the Applied Biosystems 391 PCR MATE DNA synthesizer (Applied Biosystems, Foster City, CA) using standard phosphoramidite chemistry.
2. Following synthesis, oligonucleotides are cleaved from the column using NH$_4$OH and evaporated to dryness (Savant Speedivac).
3. Oligonucleotides are phenol/chloroform extracted and divided into two Eppendorf tubes prior to ethanol precipitation.
4. Oligonucleotides are lyophilized to dryness.
5. Add 200 μL ddH$_2$O to one of the two tubes.
6. Take a 20-μL aliquot and make up to 1 mL with ddH$_2$O.
7. An Optical Density reading at 260 nm (OD$_{260}$) is measured to estimate the concentration of oligonucleotide (*see* Note 8).
8. A stock solution of 20–50 pmol/μL is made up based on the oligonucleotide concentration. Synthesis on the 40-nm scale (the lowest synthesis scale on the Applied Biosystems DNA Synthesizer) should yield a stock of 50–75 pmol/μL of a 20-mer oligonucleotide.
9. The second aliquot of oligonucleotide is stored dry at –20°C with the first aliquot. The diluted working solution may be stored at 4°C as constant freezing and thawing of the working solution may be detrimental to the stability of the oligonucleotide.
10. PCR is performed using 500 ng DNA template in a 50-μL reaction containing 5 μL 10X PCR buffer, 5 μL 10X dNTP mix, and 50 pmol each primer.
11. Use of a control primer in the same reaction tube permits a control for false negativity owing to lack of amplifiable material or a PCR failure.
12. Use of nested primers (primers designed to lie inside the first set of primers for a second round of PCR) allows greater sensitivity. In this scenario a primary amplification is performed with the outer primers (*see* Table 1).

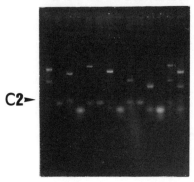

Fig. 1. Primary and nested amplification of Y chromosome specific markers. Male (M) or Female (F) DNA was amplified with a panel of markers (*see* Table 1) and electrophoresed on a 1.8% agarose gel. Lane 1, Y1,Y3 male; lane 2, Y1,Y3 female; lane 3, Y1 (nested); lane 4, no DNA; lane 5, Y2 male; lane 6, Y2 female; lane 7, Y2 (nested); lane 8, no DNA; lane 9, Y3 male; lane 10, Y3 female; lane 11, Y3 (nested); lane 12, no DNA; lane 13, Y2,Y3; lane 14, Y2,Y3 (nested). The sizes of the amplified fragments are as in Table 1. Lanes 1–6, 8–10, and 12–14 were coamplified with autosomal primers from the first exon of the rhodopsin gene ([C2] *see* Table 1).

Table 1
Sequence of Y Chromosome Specific
and Autosomal Primers[a]

Primer	Sequence	Size
Y1(+)	CTA GAC CGC AGA GGC GCC AT	239
Y1(–)	TAG TAC CCA CGC CTG CTC CG	
N1(+)	TCT GGG CCA ATG TTG TAT CC	131
N1(–)	AAG AGT CAC ATC GAA GCC GA	
Y2(+)	TCA TGG CTT GCC ACA CTC AG	321
Y2(–)	ACG CGG GCT GCG TGG TCT TT	
N2(+)	AAA GAC CAC GCA GCC CGC GT	205
N2(–)	CCC TAA GGA CTG CGC GCT AA	
Y3(+)	GTG TGG TCT CGC GAT CAG AG	185
Y3(–)	CGA TAC TTA TAA TTC GGG TA	
N3(+)	ATG GCT CTA GAG AAT CCC AG	116
N3(–)	TAA TTT CTG TGC CTC CTG GA	
C1(+)	TGG AGG AGC CAT GGT CTG GA	147
C1(–)	AGG GCA CCC AGC AGA TCA GG	
C2(+)	TTC TCC AAT GCG ACG GGT GT	80
C2(–)	ATG GAG AAC TGC CAT GGC TC	

[a]All sequences are written 5' to 3'. In each case, N1,2,3 are primers designed internally to Y1,2,3 to allow nested amplification to increase sensitivity. C1 and C2 are control primers that amplify autosomal sequences. C1 is from exon 4 of the rhodopsin gene while C2 is from exon 1 of the rhodopsin gene.

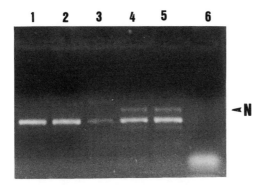

Fig. 2. Detection of mixed chimerism using nested PCR. A male recipient of a sex mismatched BMT was initially investigated using a single primer set (Y2) with C1 as a positive control. Lane 1, d 28 post-BMT; lane 2, d 56 post-BMT; lane 3, d 91 post-BMT; lane 4, d 91 post-BMT (nested); lane 5, d 171 post-BMT (nested); lane 6, negative control. The d-91 sample (lane 3) showed a faint Y-specific product. Use of nested primers (lanes 4 and 5) confirmed the presence of male (recipient) material.

13. Some 1–2 μL of this amplification reaction are subsequently used as template in a second PCR using the inner or internal primers.
14. The Y-specific PCR assay is at its most useful when the donor is female and the recipient is male, as re-emergence of recipient cells can be correlated with a reappearance of the Y signal on ethidium bromide stained gels (Fig. 2). However, this methodology is limited by its lack of quantitation and its suitability to sex mismatched transplants only. However, it is a very sensitive method of detecting minimal numbers of re-emerging cells, particularly if nested PCR is used or if Southern blot analysis is performed on amplified samples *(16)*.

3.5. PCR of Variable Number Tandem Repeat Sequences (VNTR-PCR)

A variety of VNTR markers have been adapted to the PCR format. Several parameters should be used in the judicious choice of VNTR markers. The markers should generally amplify loci of less than 2 kb in length, as it has been reported that differential amplification occurs with alleles longer than 2 kb. Markers should also be chosen that do not have a high GC content as *Taq* polymerase does not amplify these regions very efficiently. Finally, markers should have high polymorphism information content (PIC) values so that virtually all donor recipient pairs can be analyzed with a suitable primer panel. With these criteria in mind, the following VNTRs are suitable for PCR analysis and chimerism studies *(5,8,17)*: 33.6 from chromosome 1; 33.4 which is unassigned; 3'HVR from the β globin gene on 16p13.3; YNZ 22 from chromosome 17p13.3; and H-ras from the Harvey ras proto-oncogene locus on chromosome 11p15.5. This panel of minisatellite/VNTRs primer sequences is listed in Table 2.

Table 2
Sequence of PCR Primers, Forward (F) and Reverse (R), for Amplification of VNTR Loci[a]

Locus		Primer sequence	LSO sequence
33.4	F	ATG GGG GAC CGG GCC AGA CC	GGG GCA CCC ACA ATC TGG GGC CAC AGG A
	R	CCA GGA GGC CAC CAG AAC CT	
33.6	F	TGT GAG TAG AGG AGA CCT CAC	CCT CCA GCC CTC CTC CAG CCC T
	R	AAA GAC CAC AGA GTG AGG AGC	
YNZ 22	F	GGT CGA AGA GTG AAG TGC ACA G	TTG CTT CTG TAA GGG AGG GTC TCA CAG
	R	GCC CCA TGT ATC TTG TGC AGT G	
HVR	F	AGT CCC ACC TGC AGG AAA AGG GTG	GTG TCG CTG TTC CCC CCG TGT CGC TGT T
	R	GTC ACT TGG GAT TGA TGC TGT GC	
H RAS	F	TTG GGG GAG AGC TAG CAG GG	CAC TCC CCC TTC TCT CCA GGG GAC GCC A
	R	CCT CCT GCA CAG GGT CAC CT	

[a]The DNA sequence of the locus specific oligonucleotides (LSO) is also shown.

1. Amplifications should be performed in 50-μL reactions containing 1X PCR buffer, 200 μ*M* each dNTP, 12.5 pmol each primer, and 250 ng template DNA.
2. For VNTRs 33.6 and H-ras, the cycling conditions are 94°C for 1 min, 64°C for 1 min, and 72°C for 4 min for 30 cycles of amplification; for HVR and YNZ 22, the extension step at 72°C is extended to 5 min while for 33.4, the annealing temperature is reduced to 60°C.
3. Following amplification, 20 μL of each amplified product is mixed with 2 μL of 10X loading buffer and electrophoresed on a 1% agarose gel.
4. Following electrophoresis, the DNA is transferred to the membrane of choice for hybridization analysis. Prehybridization conditions will vary depending on the membrane used.
5. Hybridization is performed using an oligonucleotide probe or locus specific oligonucleotide (LSO), which is complimentary to the repeat unit. The repeat unit length varies from locus to locus; e.g., for 33.6 the repeat unit length is 11 bases and so a 22-mer oligonucleotide containing 2 complimentary tandem copies of the 11-mer core is used as a probe (*see* Table 2). For the other markers, the repeat unit length is longer (17–28 bases) and an oligonucleotide probe is designed to compliment either 1 or 1.5 repeat units
6. The bound DNA is hybridized with the appropriate 3' α^{32}P-labeled LSO for 2 h at 65°C and washed to a stringency of 1X SSC 0.1% SDS at the hybridization temperature.
7. The membrane is placed in an X-ray cassette with intensifying screens and exposed to autoradiographic film at –70°C. A radioactive signal can be detected after 2 h of hybridization, although overnight exposure is probably necessary for the detection of minor cell populations. Estimations of the sensitivity of this technique vary from 0.1 to 1% for detection of the minor cell population, depending on the primer pair used.

3.6. PCR of Short Tandem Repeats (STR-PCR) (see Notes 9–12)

The use of STR sequences in the assessment of chimerism has proved to be a highly sensitive and robust technique. Sensitivity is increased by addition of a radioactively labeled nucleotide in the PCR ("Hot" PCR). As In VNTR PCR, a panel of primers is initially used to screen donor and recipient for informative polymorphisms. The STRs that we routinely use are:

- INT 2: A dinucleotide repeat polymorphism from the int 2 proto-oncogene on chromosome 11q13.
- ACPP: A tetranucleotide repeat from the 3' noncoding region of the prostatic acid phosphatase gene on chromosome 3q21.
- CYP 19: A tetranucleotide repeat polymorphism from the human aromatase cytochrome P450 gene on chromosome 15q21.
- IGF 1: A dinucleotide repeat from the insulin growth-factor gene on chromosome 12q22.
- vWF: A tetranucleotide repeat from the von Willebrand Factor locus on chromosome 12.

The DNA sequence of these primer pairs and their degree of polymorphism is shown in Table 3.

Table 3
Primer Sequences and Heterozygosity (HET) or Polymorphism Information Content (PIC values) of Dinucleotide and Short Tandem Repeat Markers

Locus	Sequence	Size range	HET	PIC value
INT 2	TTT CTG GGT GTG TGT CTG AAT ACA CAG TTG CTC TAA AGG GT	161–177 bp	84.6%	
ACPP	ACT GTG CCT AGC CTA TAC TT AGT GAG CCA AGA GTG CAC TA	136–156 bp		0.58
CYP19	GCA GGT ACT TTA AGT TAG CTA TTA CAG TGA GCC CAA GGT CGT	154–178 bp	91.3%	
vWF	TGT ACC TAG TTA TCT ATC CTG GTG ATG ATG ATG GAG ACA GAG	154–174 bp		0.65
IGF	GCT AGC CAG CTG GTG TTA TT ACC ACT CTG GGA GAA GGG TA	178–196 bp		0.53

1. Make up a reaction tube containing a 200-ng template: 2.5 µL DNA, 10X PCR buffer mix, 2.5 µL 10X dNTP mix, and 25–100 µ*M* dCTP (this concentration can vary for different STRs). Add ddH$_2$O to 20 µL total volume.
2. Overlay with 25 µL paraffin oil and heat to 95°C for 7 min. Reduce temperature to 80°C for 10 min.
3. Add the following in a 5-µL solution ("Hot start procedure"): 1 U *Taq* polymerase, 25 pmol each primer, and 1 µCi α^{32}P dCTP at 3000 Ci/mmol (Amersham).
4. PCR is performed using the following cycling parameters for 30 cycles: 94°C for 1 min (for primers CYP 19 and INT 2, this time is extended to 1.4 min), 55°C for 1 min (for primer vWF, this time is extended to 1.4 min; for primer ACPP, the annealing temperature is raised to 60°C), and 72°C for 1.2 min (*see* Note 13).
5. After 30 cycles of amplification, 2.5 µL of product are mixed with an equal volume of formamide tracking dye and loaded on an 8% denaturing polyacrylamide sequencing gel.
6. To make up a sequencing gel: Mix 30 mL of the 20% acrylamide solution and 45 mL urea solution.
7. Add 400 µL ammonium persulfate and 75 µL TEMED immediately prior to pouring the gel to aid in polymerization. Make sure to mix well prior to pouring to ensure even polymerization of the gel matrix.
8. Pour gel taking care to avoid bubbles and allow gel to set for 30 min to 1 h depending on ambient room temperature.
9. Set up gel in sequencing apparatus. Make sure to use same TBE stock in electrophoresis buffer to ensure equal concentration of ions.
10. Electrophorese gel at a constant power (35 W and approx 1,500 V). The xylene cyanol front runs at approx 75 bases on an 8% gel allowing estimation of the time required for adequate separation of di or tetranucleotide repeats.

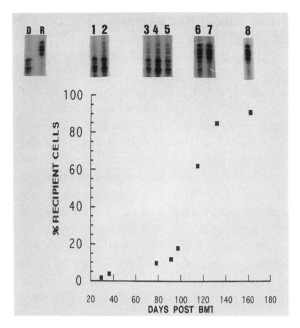

Fig. 3. STR-PCR in the detection of MC. D, donor; R, recipient. Lane 1, d 29 post-BMT; lane 2, d 36 post-BMT; lane 3, d 75 post-BMT; lane 4, d 91 post-BMT; lane 5, d 100 post-BMT; lane 6, d 114 post-BMT; lane 7, d 131 post-BMT; lane 8, d 161 post-BMT. Donor and recipient are maximally informative for nonoverlapping heterozygote alleles. Operator (not shown) shown shared one allele with the lower allele of the donor but showed a distinctly different second allele from donor or recipient. While initial levels of recipient cells were low (<10%), subsequent re-emergence of recipient cells occurred after d 100 leading to graft rejection at d 191.

11. Following electrophoresis, gels are dried down and subjected to autoradiography. Efficient labeling of the PCR template can result in a strong signal in 2–3 h if the dried gel is placed in an X-ray cassette with intensifying screens at −70°C. This technique allows detection of the minor cell population at levels of 0.01–0.1%.

An example of the use of STR-PCR is shown in Fig. 3. Donor and recipient were found to be informative for the dinucleotide repeat IGF1. As the CA and GT bands of the microsatellite migrate with different mobilities owing to the denaturing properties of the gel, a homozygote will yield two bands and a heterozygote 4 bands. The strand containing CA will be labeled more strongly as Cytosine is the radioactive nucleotide in the reaction. As seen from Fig. 3, both donor and recipient show nonoverlapping heterozygote profiles. Analysis of early posttransplant samples reveals predominantly donor hemopoiesis but there is a sudden rise in recipient cells around d 100 post-BMT. This sudden rise, which is termed progressive mixed chimerism, preceded subsequent graft rejection on d 191.

Recently, several methods have been developed to allow nonradioactive detection of STR alleles. Use of chemiluminescence techniques allows detection of amplified alleles after blotting of acrylamide onto nylon membranes and probing using the ECL oligonucleotide labeling and detection system (Amersham, UK). Alternatively, STR primers may be labeled with a fluorophore and detected after electrophoresis on a Model 373 DNA sequencer (Applied Biosystems). The principle of this electrophoresis system is that an argon laser excites the fluorophore labeled product at a particular wavelength and allows detection of the fluorescent product. Use of different fluorophores allows multiple markers to be electrophoresed in the same lane of a gel. Either of these systems could allow chimerism studies in large numbers of samples.

The ability to assess archival material using STR markers has allowed retrospective studies to be performed and has allowed access to pretransplant material from stored hematological slides or paraffin-embedded material. The use of serial studies with polymorphic markers (either STRs or VNTRs) allows direct comparison of donor and recipient profiles, and thus semiquantitative data is available on the kinetics of engraftment. This may be important in assessing the likelihood of recurrence of disease in certain patients.

Chimerism studies are useful in assessing the outcome of the transplant procedure. Studies in recipients of T-cell depleted grafts have indicated that this group contains higher numbers of mixed chimeras when compared to patients receiving unmanipulated bone marrow. In Chronic Myeloid Leukemia, T-cell depletion, mixed chimerism, and leukemia relapse are linked. Studies of separated cell populations indicate that mixed T-cell chimerism is associated with a higher level of minimal residual disease and a higher risk of leukemic relapse *(16)*. CML is one of the few diseases where a defined graft vs leukemia effect can be seen and clinical use of donor leukocyte infusions is now an important therapeutic option for relapsed CML. Chimerism studies are important in monitoring the immunotherapeutic response.

In aplastic anemia, a large laboratory based study by our group for the European Bone Marrow and Blood Transplant working party on Severe Aplastic Anemia indicates that patients with rising levels of recipient cells (progressive mixed chimerism) are at a higher risk of graft rejection. Chimerism studies, while not as sensitive as Minimal Residual Disease studies using either disease specific or clonality markers, compare favorably with these techniques in the majority of transplant recipients. In situations where there is no specific marker of disease relapse, chimerism studies may be of particular value.

PCR of VNTRs or STRs is the most reliable technique at present for assessment of chimerism post-BMT. A single bone marrow or peripheral blood smear can provide enough genetic material for 5–20 analyses. As chimerism studies use nondisease specific markers, the use of single timepoint studies is of little value either in understanding the kinetics of chimerism or in patient management. Serial studies using peripheral blood or bone marrow are necessary if we are to understand the kinetics of engraftment, graft rejection, or leukemia relapse either early or late post transplant *(17)*. The robustness of this technique may allow it to become the first choice in testing patients at risk and providing data to referring clinicians.

4. Notes

1. This may vary depending on the source of *Taq* polymerase used.
2. For any PCR-based study, access to DNA is more straightforward. As PCR is a more robust technique than Southern blotting, initial starting material can be of lower molecular weight and of less high quality. However, whereas there are several "quick and dirty" methods of isolating DNA for "once off" PCR, chimerism studies require serial analysis of DNA samples. Thus, a technique is required that yields DNA of sufficient quality for repeated use. Routine analysis in our laboratory involves the isolation of DNA from stored nonstained nonfixed hematological slides *(17)*. This allows prospective as well as retrospective studies to be performed and allows easy access to material from collaborating centers. A standard bone marrow or peripheral blood smear will yield 1–10 µg DNA, which is sufficient for multiple analyses.
3. A separate blade should be used for each sample to avoid crosscontamination, and this procedure should take place in a laminar air hood as an added precaution against contamination.
4. Isolation of material from stained slides is less reliable, particularly if they are also coverslipped. Soaking of slides overnight in xylene as is standard for extraction of DNA from formalin-fixed paraffin-embedded material can make them more amenable to subsequent extraction.
5. When performing chimerism studies by PCR analysis, it is necessary to exclude potential sources of contamination. One potential source of contamination is the operator, so it is advisable to include an operator control with each chimerism study. The easiest source of operator DNA is from a buccal wash and this provides adequate material for multiple analyses.
6. In some cases, paraffin-embedded material may be the only material available for analysis for deducing the pretransplant profile of the recipient. Such archival material may have DNA that has been damaged by the fixing process; it has been noted that samples of this kind may be difficult to amplify with primers that give a product in access of 400–500 bp. However, DNA from paraffin-embedded material is particularly suited to PCR of STRs or microsatellites as the size of product generated is 100–200 bp. A standard paraffin-embedded protocol *(18)* allows access to this material.
7. In any PCR-based assay system, the following precautions should be taken to avoid contamination.
   a. All scraping of slide material should be undertaken in a laminar flow hood and each sample processed individually with a separate sterile scalpel blade.

  b. Sample preparation and PCR amplification should be performed in different areas.

  c. Plugged tips can be used to avoid aerosol-borne contamination.

  d. Buffers can be incubated with restriction enzymes that cut within the amplified fragment before amplification to ensure that any contaminating material does not act as a template for PCR. Restriction enzymes can subsequently be heat killed to ensure no interference with PCR.

  e. Other more stringent contamination measures such as the use of positive displacement pipets, UV irradiation of solutions prior to PCR, or the use of the Uracil N Glycosylase PCR carryover prevention kit (Roche) can also be performed.

 8. The following formula can be used to estimate oligonucleotide concentration, based on the OD reading at 260 nm.

$$1\ OD_{260}\ U = 33\ \mu g\ \text{for an oligonucleotide}$$

$$OD/\mu L \times 33 \times 10^6/330 \times \text{no. of bases} = pmol/\mu L = \mu M$$

 9. STR-PCR. Depending on the number of reactions being performed, a master mix should be made up of *Taq* polymerase, primers and radioactively labeled dCTP just prior to addition. Thus the minimum number of manipulations can be carried out with radioactively labeled material.

 10. STR-PCR. The loci described were chosen owing to their high information content and relative robustness. There are many other STR loci described in the literature that are also suitable for chimerism studies.

 11. STR-PCR. STR-PCR can also be performed by labeling one of the amplification primers with $\gamma^{32}P$ dATP using polynucleotide kinase. This allows labeling of one strand so homozygotes appear as a single band and heterozygotes as a doublet (*see* ref. *19* for detailed description). However, while this methodology is useful for screening a large number of DNA samples with a single marker, it is more time consuming and wasteful of isotope if a panel of markers is being used to screen small numbers of samples, as is the case in typing donor recipient pairs and assessing posttransplant chimerism. In this case, the use of a single isotopic label that can be incorporated into a reaction is more generally applicable.

 12. STR PCR. The use of the "hot start procedure" avoids the problems of nonspecific amplification, which usually occurs owing to primer annealing of oligonucleotide to target at low temperatures below the expected melting temperature of the primer target duplex. Addition of the primers with polymerase and radioactive dCTP after initial denaturation at an elevated temperature avoids this potential problem.

 13. Primer dilution curves and magnesium buffer optima studies should be performed for any new oligonucleotide pair. It is recommended that this is done using both "cold" (no radioactive dCTP added) and "hot" (radioactive dCTP added in the dNTP buffer) PCR assay conditions, as differences have occasionally been seen (Lawler, unpublished). The timing of these annealing and extension times may vary depending on the type of thermal cycler so optimum annealing and extending times should be assessed using control material. The concentration of cold dCTP in the dNTP solution is low owing to the addition of radioactive dCTP to the PCR.

References

1. Blazar, B. R., Orr, H. T., Arthur, D. C., Kersey, J. H., and Filipovich, A. H. (1985) Restriction fragment length polymorphisms as markers of engraftment in allogeneic marrow transplantation. *Blood*, **66**, 1436–1444.
2. Knowlton, R. G., Brown, V. A., Braman, J. C., Barker, D., Schumm, J. W., Murray, C., Takuorian, T., Ritz, J., and Donis-Keller, H. (1986) Use of highly polymorphic DNA probes for genotypic analysis following bone marrow transplantation. *Blood*, **68**, 378–385.
3. Lawler, M., McCann, S. R., Conneally, E., and Humphries, P. (1989) Chimaerism following allogeneic bone marrow transplantation; detection of residual host cells using the polymerase chain reaction. *Br. J. Haematol.* **73**, 205–210.
4. Socie, G., Landman, J., Gluckman, E., Devergie, A., Raynal, B., Esperou-Bourdeau, H., and Brison, O. (1992) Short term study of chimaerism after bone marrow transplantation for severe aplastic anaemia. *Br. J. Haematol.* **80**, 391–398.
5. Uggozoli, L., Yam, P., Petz, L. D., Felttera, G. B., Champlin, R. E., Forman, S. J., Koyal, D., and Wallace, R. B. (1991) Amplification by the polymerase chain reaction of hypervariable regions of the human genome for evaluation of chimerism after bone marrow transplantation. *Blood* **77**, 1607–1615.
6. Weber, J. I. and May, P. E. (1989) Abundant class of DNA polymorphisms which can be typed using the polymerase chain reaction. *Am. J. Hum. Genet.* **44**, 388–396.
7. Lawler, M., Humphries, P., and McCann, S. R. (1991) Evaluation of mixed chimerism by in vitro amplification of dinucleotide repeat sequences using the polymerase chain reaction. *Blood* **77**, 2504–2514.
8. Mackinnon, S., Barnett, L., Bourhis, J. H., Black, P., Heller, G. O., and Reilly, R. J. (1992) Myeloid and lymphoid chimerism after T cell-depleted bone marrow transplantation, evaluation of conditioning regimen using the polymerase chain reaction to amplify human minisatellite regions of genomic DNA. *Blood* **80**, 3235–3241.
9. Roux, E., Helg, C., Chapuis, B., Jeannet, M., and Roosnek, E. (1992) Evolution of mixed chimerism after allogeneic bone marrow transcription as determined on granulocytes and mononuclear cells by the polymerase chain reaction. *Blood* **79**, 2775–2783.
10. Van Leuwen, J. E. M., Van Tol, M. J. D., Bodzinga, B. G., Wijner, J. Th., van der Keor, M., Jooster, A. M., Tanke, H. J., Vossen, J. M., and Meera Khan, P. (1991) Detection of mixed chimaerism in flow sorted cell subpopulations by PCR amplified VNTR markers after allogeneic bone marrow transplantation. *Br. J. Haematol.* **79**, 218–225.
11. Roux, E., Abdi, K., Speiser, D., Helg, C., Chapuis, B., Jeannet, M., and Roosnek, E. (1993) Characterisation of mixed chimerism in patients with chronic myeloid leukemia transplanted with T cell-depleted marrow, involvement of different hematopoietic lineages before and after relapse. *Blood* **81**, 243–248.
12. Mercier, B., Gaucher, C., Feugeas, O., and Mazurier, C. (1990) Direct PCR from whole blood, without DNA extraction. *Nucleic Acids Res.* **18**, 5908.
13. Bell, G. I., Karam, J. H., and Rutter, W. J. (1981) Polymorphic DNA region adjacent to the 5' end of the human insulin gene. *Proc. Natl. Acad. Sci. USA* **78**, 5759–5763.

14. Sambrook, J., Fritsch, E. F., and Maniatis, T. (1989) *Molecular Cloning: A Laboratory Manual*, 2nd ed., Cold Spring Harbor Laboratory, Cold Spring Harbor, NY.
15. Socie, G., Gluckman, E., Raynal, B., Petit, T., Landman, J., Devergie, A., and Brison, O. (1993) Bone marrow transplantation for Fanconi anemia using low dose cyclophosphamide-thoracoabdominal irradiation as conditioning regimen, chimerism study by the polymerase chain reaction. *Blood* **82,** 2249–2256.
16. Mackinnon, S., Barnett, I., Heller, G., and O Reilly, R. J. (1994) Minimal residual disease is more common in patients who have mixed T cell chimerism after Bone Marrow transplantation for Chronic Myelogenous Leukemia. *Blood* **83,** 3409–3416.
17. McCann, S. R. and Lawler, M. (1993) Mixed chimerism; detection and significance following BMT. *Bone Marrow Transplant* **11,** 91–94.
18. Fey, M. F., Pilkington, S. P., Summers, C., and Wainscoat, J. S. (1987) Molecular diagnosis of haematological disorders using DNA from stored bone marrow slides. *Br. J. Haematol.* **67,** 489–492.
19. Shibata, D. (1994) Preparation of nucleic acids from archival material, in *PCR: The Polymerase Chain Reaction* (Mullis, K. B., Ferre, F., and Gibbs, R. A., eds.), Birkhauser, Boston, pp. 47–54.
20. Litt, M. (1991) PCR of TG Microsatellites, in *PCR: A Practical Approach* (McPherson, M. J., Quirke, P., and Taylor, G. R., eds.), IRL, Oxford, pp. 85–100.

II

SOLID TUMORS

10

Identification
of Mutations in the Retinoblastoma Gene

Annette Hogg

1. Introduction

Mutations in the retinoblastoma gene (RB1) predispose to the formation of ocular tumors. Following the cloning of RB1 in 1986 *(1)*, polymorphic restriction enzyme sites within RB1 were used to "track" the mutant gene within affected families using linkage analysis *(2,3)*. This approach, however, was unsuitable for most retinoblastoma (Rb) patients because only 16% have a family history of Rb *(4)*. In recent years, it has become possible to detect mutations in nucleic acids. The ability to detect mutations in RB1 has important implications for Rb patients because it means that individuals predisposed to Rb but with no previous family history of the disease can now be screened for mutations.

Single-strand conformation polymorphism analysis (SSCP) *(5)* has a number of advantages compared to other mutation detection techniques for the analysis of RB1. SSCP is simple, requires a minimum number of manipulations, and involves the use of relatively safe chemicals. In addition, it is ideal for screening large, complex genes, such as RB1, which contains 27 exons *(6)*. One potential disadvantage of SSCP is that the sensitivity decreases when DNA molecules longer than 250 bp are analyzed. The inability to detect mutations in large molecules is a potential problem if cDNA is analyzed but this approach probably is not suitable for most RB1 mutations. The analysis of RB1 cDNA appears to be unsuitable because mutations that have been detected in RB1 genomic DNA often do not produce detectable levels of mutant RB1 mRNA in lymphocytes *(7–9)*. The reason for the lack of mutant RB1 mRNA in lymphocytes is unknown but the instability of mRNA transcripts which contain premature stop codons (which are the most common inactivating mutation in the RB1 gene) may be responsible *(10–12)*. For this reason, an exon-by-exon analysis of RB1 often is required.

From: *Methods in Molecular Medicine, Molecular Diagnosis of Cancer*
Edited by: F. E. Cotter Humana Press Inc., Totowa, NJ

The SSCP technique is based on the observation that the migration of single stranded DNA molecules in a nondenaturing polyacrylamide gel is sequence-dependent. The conformation of a single-stranded (SS) DNA molecule in solution depends on intrastrand hydrogen bonding as well as base stacking. Thus, the conformation of SS DNA molecules can be altered by point mutations, deletions (Fig. 1) and insertions and this can change their mobility in a gel when compared to a normal DNA fragment.

In order to detect mutations in RB1, it is necessary to produce large quantities of DNA for mutation analysis using the polymerase chain reaction (PCR) *(13)*. Oligonucleotide primers located in the introns, within 50 bp of each exon, have been designed for the RB1 gene *(14)*. In most cases, the PCR-amplified exon is too long for analysis using SSCP and appropriate restriction enzyme are used, therefore, to produce fragments <250 bp (or as close as possible). Finally, the DNA is denatured and electophoresed on a nondenaturing polyacrylamide "SSCP" gel. The nature of the mutation can be determined by sequence analysis of the PCR product that generated the aberrantly migrating DNA.

2. Materials

2.1. General Reagents

1. MilliQ purified and autoclaved water.
2. Neutral loading dye: 0.25% bromophenol blue, 0.25% xylene cyanol, 15% Ficoll (Type 400).
3. 10X *Taq* polymerase buffer: 500 mM KCl, 100 mM Tris-HCl, pH 9.0, 0.1% gelatin (w/v), 1% Triton X-100, 15 mM MgCl$_2$.
4. dNTP (deoxynucleotide) mix: 2.0 mM dATP, 2.0 mM dCTP, 2.0 mM dGTP, 2.0 mM dTTP.
5. TAE agarose gel running buffer: 0.04M Tris-acetate, 1.0 mM EDTA, 0.5 μg/mL ethidium bromide (50X TAE: 242 g Tris base, 57.1 mL glacial acetic acid, 100 mL 0.5M EDTA, pH 8.0).
6. STE: 10 mM Tris-HCl, pH 8.0, 1 mM EDTA, 0.1M NaCl, pH 8.0.

2.2. Sample Preparation

1. Blood lysis buffer: 0.075M NaCl, 0.024M EDTA.
2. Cell lysis buffer: 100 mM NaCl, 10 mM EDTA, 100 mM Tris-HCl, pH 8.0.
3. 10% SDS (sodium dodecylsulfate).
4. Phosphate-buffered saline A (PBSA).
5. 1M Tris-HCl, pH 8.0.
6. TE: 10 mM Tris-HCl, pH 8.0, 1 mM EDTA, pH 8.0.
7. TE-saturated phenol: Equilibrate water saturated phenol with 1M Tris-HCl, pH 8.0 and add hydroxyquinolone to 0.1%.
8. 0.1% Nonidet P 40.
9. 3M Sodium acetate, pH 5.2.
10. Proteinase K: 20 mg/mL.

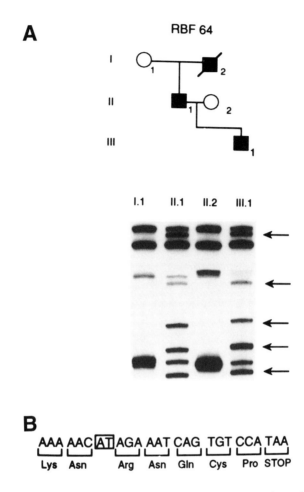

Fig. 1. SSCP analysis of exon 3 from family RBF 64. DNA from four individuals from family RBF 64 was analyzed using SSCP. DNA from affected individuals II.1 and III.1 formed several bands on the SSCP gel (arrows) that were absent from the unaffected individuals, I.1 and II.2. The DNA was sequenced and a 2 bp deletion 106 bp from the 5' end of exon 3 was identified in individuals II.1 and III.1. The consequence of the mutation is shown in **(B)**. The deleted bases (boxed) generated a shift in the reading frame producing a stop codon 15 bp further downstream.

2.3. Single-Strand Conformation Polymorphism Analysis (SSCP)

1. SSCP dNTP mix: 2.0 m*M* dATP, 2.0 m*M* dTTP, 2.0 m*M* dGTP. 0.2 m*M* dCTP.
2. [α-^{32}P] dCTP: 3000Ci/m*M*.
3. 40% acrylamide (1:20 *bis*): 40% Acrylamide w/v: *N,N'*-methylene bisacrylamide at a ratio of 1:20.

4. Glycerol.
5. 10X Tris-borate electrophoresis buffer (TBE): $0.9M$ Tris base, $0.9M$ boric acid, 25 mM EDTA.
6. Polyacrylamide gel loading dye mix: 95% formamide, 20 mM EDTA, 0.05% bromophenol blue, 0.05% xylene cyanol.

2.4. Equipment

1. Thermocycler.
2. Sequencing gel running apparatus.
3. Agarose gel running apparatus.
4. Gel drier.
5. Centrifuge.

3. Methods

The following procedure outlines the techniques required for the analysis of mutations in the RB1 gene. First, DNA is prepared from blood samples or alternatively, whole blood can be used directly in PCR. The latter method is faster, but, occasionally, inhibitors, such as hemoglobin, may interfere with the PCR, resulting in a low yield of product (*see later*).

3.1. Preparation of DNA from Lymphocytes

1. Collect 10-mL blood samples in lithium heparin anticoagulant tubes.
2. Mix each 10-mL sample with 20 mL of sterile, cold distilled water to lyse the red cells.
3. Centrifuge at 1300g for 15 min, remove the supernatant and resuspend the pellet, containing the white blood cells, in 30 mL of 0.1% Nonidet P 40 in order to lyse the cell membrane but not the nuclear membrane.
4. Centrifuge at 1300g for 15 min, remove the supernatant, and resuspend the nuclei in 5 mL of blood lysis buffer. Add SDS to a final concentration of 1.0%.
5. Add proteinase K to a final concentration of 100 μg/mL and incubate overnight at 37°C or for 2 h at 60°C in order to digest the cellular proteins.
6. After proteinase K digestion, extract the DNA with phenol:chloroform using the upper end of a 10-mL pipet to prevent shearing the DNA.
7. Add to the final upper phase 2.5 vol of ethanol and 1/10 vol of 3M sodium acetate pH 5.2. Genomic DNA should precipitate immediately and be visible as a stringy white mass. Collect the DNA by spooling using a glass Pasteur pipet. Wash the DNA in 70% ethanol to remove excess salts and resuspend in 2 mL of TE. If, after resuspension in TE, the solution is white and cloudy the proteinase K treatment (*see the preceding*) should be repeated to remove undigested cellular proteins.
8. Remove an aliquot from the DNA and dilute to 1:20 in distilled water. Measure the absorbance of the DNA solution, at 260 nm, in a glass cuvet in a spectrophotometer.

3.2. Preparation of DNA from Whole Blood

Although DNA for PCR amplification can be prepared by standard phenol-chloroform extraction, as described earlier, a simple and rapid procedure can also be used for whole blood, as follows (*see* Note 1).

1. Collect blood samples in lithium heparin anticoagulant tubes.
2. Add 2 µL of whole blood to 5 µL of 10X *Taq* polymerase buffer/5 µL of dNTP mix and adjust the volume to 50 µL with water.
3. Lyse the cells by performing three successive PCR cycles, each consisting of 3 min at 95°C and 3 min at 65°C.

3.3. PCR

Oligonucleotide primers are used to amplify RB1 DNA for analysis using PCR. These oligonucleotide primers were designed using the sequence of the coding region of RB1, together with approx 200 bp of the introns flanking each exon, reported by McGee et al. *(6)*. Primers are deliberately located within intron sequences to allow the analysis of splice sites, detection of activated cryptic splice sites or new splice sites, and analysis of branchpoints that are usually 30–50 bp upstream from the splice acceptor site. Details of oligonucle-otide primer pairs designed to amplify exons 1–26, the coding region of exon 27, the 5' promoter region and the 3' poly-A signal sequence of RB1 are listed in Table 1. All of the sets of primers listed in Table 1 give a single PCR product when electrophoresed on 1.5% agarose/TAE gels.

Some general points to consider when performing PCR are in Notes 2–6.

1. Add to a PCR tube on ice the following: 100 ng of purified DNA or 2 µL of whole blood (*see* Note 7), 50 pm of each PCR primer (for the particular exon being analyzed), 5 µL of 10X *Taq* polymerase buffer/5 µL of dNTP mix or SSCP dNTP mix (*see* Section 3.4.) and adjust to a final volume of 50 µL with distilled water. Overlay with 30 µL of mineral oil.
2. Program the thermocycler to carry out a 10-min denaturation step at 95°C followed by an incubation at 65°C. After the thermocycler begins to cool to 65°C, add 1 U of *Taq* polymerase through the oil. The addition of *Taq* polymerase at 65°C (which is higher than the annealing temperature of the primers) increases the specificity of the reaction. The time allowed for the incubation at 65°C will depend on the length of time required for the addition of the *Taq* polymerase. After the addition of the *Taq* polymerase, perform 30 PCR cycles consisting of an initial denaturation step at 96°C for 0.5 min followed by an annealing step at a temperature optimal for the particular primer pair (*see* Table 1) for 0.5 min and an extension step at 72°C for 1 min.

3.4. SSCP

DNA for SSCP analysis is generated by PCR amplification using the primers listed in Table 1. Many of the oligonucleotide primers listed in Table 1 yield PCR products that are longer than 250 bp, which is considered the upper

Table 1
Details of the Oligonucleotide Primers for Amplification and Analysis Using SSCP of the 27 Exons of RB1[a]

Oligo	Location	Sequence	Temp, °C	Full size, bp	5' Intron	3' Intron	RE	Cut size, bp
6007	RB 5 × Pro	GATCCCAAAAGGCCAGCAAGTGTCT	62[b]	570			SmaI	230
6008	RB 3 × Pro	TCAACGTCCCCTGAGAAAAACCGGA					BspHI	176/164
9691	RB 5 × 1	CGTGCGGCGCGTGTCCT	62[b]	307	67	103	DdeI	153
9692	RB 3 × 1	ACCCGGCCCCTGGCGAGGAC						154
10143	RB 5 × 2	GTTCTTTTTCACAGTAGTGTTATGTG	60	409	105	177	HpaI	214
10142	RB 3 × 2	CGTGCCGGCCTCAAACATTTTTAA						191
8202	RB 5 × 3	GCCATCAGAAGGATGTGTTACAA	58	477	150	211	AluI	243
8201	RB 3 × 3	GGACACAAACTGCTACCTCTTAAAG						234
8203	RB 5 × 4	CCTTCCAAAGGATATAGTAGTGATTTG	58	445	133	192	RsaI	269
8204	RB 3 × 4	CCAGGAAGCATTCAGAATGCATATT						176
8206	RB 5 × 5	GAAGACTAATTGAGAGGATTAACTG	58	488	216	233	AflIII	218
8205	RB 3 × 5	TGTCCTGAATCAATTCCACCTTATT					TaqI	142/128
8208	RB 5 × 6	GAAACACCCAAAAGATATATCTGG	58	326	85	173	AluI	179
8207	RB 3 × 6	CCAAGGTGTTTCTAGTACCAG						147
7090	RB 5 × 7	ACTCTACCCTGCGATTTTCTCTCAT	60	430	76	243	RsaI	193/176
7091	RB 3 × 7	CTTCTTGTCTCCCAAACCTCCATTTG						61

20085	RB 5 × 8	GACCTAAGTTATAGTTAGAATACTTC	55	316	81	92	TaqI	202
20084	RB 3 × 8	CATGCTCATAACAAAAGAAGTAAA						114
7095	RB 5 × 9	TGCATGGGGATTGACACCTCTAAC	60	316	106	132	EcoRI	171
7094	RB 3 × 9	CTACTTGGCTAGATTCTTCTTGGGC						145
10145	RB 5 × 10	TCTGTACCTCACTTTAGATAGACC	60	492	170	212	BglII	225/218
10144	RB 3 × 10	CTGTTATAGGACACACAATTCAC					HinfI	49
11289	RB 5 × 11	GACAACAGAAGCATTATACTGC	55	294	90	126	MboII	163
11290	RB 3 × 11	CCTGGCCTTCAATATATATTTCT						131
9987	RB 5 × 12	CCACAGTCTTATTTGAGGGAATG	60	465	146	231	BclI	198
9986	RB 3 × 12	GGTGAGCAAGGCAAATAGGTAAA					RsaI	162/105
5528	RB 5 × 13	TAATAGGGTTTTTAGTTGTACTGT	60	570	220	233	EcoRI	232
5529	RB 3 × 13	AATTTCTACAATGGCTATGTGTTCC					HinfI	225/113
13679	RB 5 × 14	CTAAAATAGCAGGCTCTTATTTTC	58	212	42	113		
13680	RB 3 × 14	ATCTTGATGCCTGACCTCCTGAT						
11293	RB 5 × 15	ATTCAATGCTGACACAAATAAGGTT	55	361	70	80	NdeI	209
11294	RB 3 × 16	TTCTCCTTAACCTCACACTATCC						152
20877	RB 5 × 17	ACTTCCAAAAAATACCTAGCTCAAG	55	315	69	49	DraI	179
23728	RB 3 × 17	TTTGTTAGCCATATGCACATGAATG						139
10604	RB 5 × 18	ATGTACCTGGGAAAATTATGCT	58	221	59	43	BclI	113
10603	RB 3 × 18	CTATTTGCAGTTTGATGGTCAAC						108

(continued)

Table 1 (continued)
Details of the Oligonucleotide Primers for Amplification and Analysis Using SSCP of the 27 Exons of RB1[a]

Oligo	Location	Sequence	Temp, °C	Full size, bp	5' Intron	3' Intron	RE	Cut size, bp
17294	RB 5 × 19	TATCTGGGTGTACAACCTTGAAGTG	62	349	223	116	MluI	218
9440	RB 3 × 19	CACAGAGATATTAAGTGACTTGCCC						131
9438	RB 5 × 20	TTCTCTCGGGGGAAAGAAAAGAGTGG	60	350	153	151	HpaII or MspI	177
14928	RB 3 × 20	AGTTAACAAGTAAGTAGGGAGGAGA						73
9436	RB 5 × 21	GACTTTCAAAACTGAGCTCAGTATGG	58	363	148	88	NdeI	191
17296	RB 3 × 21	GGTCAGACAGAATATATGATCTC						172
9434	RB 5 × 22	GCAGCTATAATCCAAGCCTAAGAAG	60	363	193	56	BclI	210
9433	RB 3 × 22	GTTTTGGTGGACCCATTACATTAGA						153
9694	RB 5 × 23	TCTAATGTAATGGGTCCACCAAAAC	58	420	62	194	BspNI	186
9695	RB 3 × 23	CATCTTGCGTTGCTTAAGTCGTAAA					AluI	136/98
9696	RB 5 × 24	TAAAACTAAGAGACTAGGTGAGTAT	58	579	205	343	BstEII	235/200
9697	RB 3 × 24	TAGATTTGGGTGAGAAAAAATCTC					HindIII/ BspNI	93/50
9991	RB 5 × 25	ATTTGGTCCAATGAAGCAGAAAATT	60	382	142	97	Bsp-1286 I	198
17249	RB 3 × 25	ATGAAAGAAATTGGTATAAGCCA						184

17250	RB 5 × 26	GTCATCGAAAGCATCATAGTTACTG	60	394	86	258	NsiI	252
9992	RB 3 × 26	TGAATGTGGTCAAGCAATGTTTCAC	142					
10609	RB 5 × 27	AAGGTCCTGAGCGCCATCAGTTTGA	62	218	108	39		
10608	RB 3 × 27	GAGGTGTACACAGTGTCCACCAAGG						
10605	RB 5 × PA	GTTTTTAGGTCAAGGGCTTAC	58	375			RsaI	162
10606	RB 3 × PA	ATCTCTAGCATATAGAGCCCTT						111/102

[a]The location of each primer is shown (i.e., 5 × 1 = 5' primer for exon 1, and so on). Pro = the promoter region. PA = poly A signal sequence. The annealing temperatures for PCR amplification and the sizes of the flanking 5' and 3' introns are shown as well as restriction enzymes (RE) used to digest PCR products and sizes of the resultant fragments. Both the promoter region and exon 1 required 10% DMSO in the PCR reaction.

[b]Primers 11293 and 11294 amplify 80 bp of intron sequence between exons 15 and 16.

limit for fragment length for SSCP analysis. Therefore, it is necessary to digest the products with appropriate restriction enzymes (Table 1) prior to analysis. Finally, the double-stranded (DS) DNA is denatured and electrophoresed on a "nondenaturing" polyacrylamide gel containing 10% glycerol, which acts as a mild denaturant. Although the PCR product is denatured by heating to 95°C and cooled on ice prior to loading on the gel, DS DNA still can be visualized. However, SS DNA is sufficiently abundant to produce an intense signal after just an overnight exposure of the resultant autoradiograph. Electrophoresis of an undenatured sample enables the position of the DS DNA on the gel to be determined, making it easy to identify which are the SS DNA molecules. SS DNA from individual exons will not always produce only two bands. Often three or four SS DNA species will be seen and are presumed to represent different conformations of the same SS DNA molecule. Some SS DNA bands may be more intense than others, indicating that some conformations may be favored more than others or that more than one species is migrating to the same position.

3.4.1. Production of DNA for SSCP Analysis

In order to visualize the DNA after analysis on polyacrylamide gels, radiolabeled dCTP is added to the PCR reaction mix. The concentration of "cold dCTP" in the dNTP mixture is reduced by a factor of 10-fold relative to the other dNTPs to promote incorporation of labeled dCTP.

3.4.2. PCR

Prepare the PCR reaction mixture on ice, as described in Section 2., except for the following modifications.

1. Use the SSCP dNTP mix.
2. Add 1 μL (10 μCi) of [α-^{32}P]dCTP (3000 Ci/mmol) to the PCR reaction mixture.

3.4.3. Agarose Gel Electrophoresis

1. Following amplification, remove most of the mineral oil layer from the surface of the PCR product.
2. Prepare a 1.5% agarose gel in TAE agarose gel running buffer. Add 3 μL of neutral loading dye to 5 μL of the PCR product and electrophorese until the bromophenol blue dye front, which migrates ahead of xylene cyanol, has traversed 2/3 of the gel. Load a DNA size marker, which includes DNA from 50 bp to 1 kb, on the gel to assess the sizes of the DNA.
3. Assess the quality and quantity of the DNA by placing the gels on a UV transilluminator. A single product and residual primers should be visualized. The DNA either is digested with an appropriate restriction enzyme (*see* Section 3.4.4.) or diluted as described in Section 3.4.5., if it already is <250 bp long.

3.4.4. Restriction Enzyme Digestion of PCR Products

In order to digest PCR products, remove 15 µL of the amplified DNA (Section 3.4.2.), from beneath the oil and incubate it overnight with 8 U of the appropriate restriction enzymes (Table 1) at 37°C (65°C for *Taq* 1 and 50°C for *Bcl* 1). In order to check that the DNA is digested, add 5 µL of TE and 3 µL of neutral loading dye to 5 µL of the digested product and electrophorese it in a 1.5% agarose gel (*see* Section 3.4.3.).

3.4.5. Sample Preparation

Remove a 5-µL aliquot of the PCR product from (Section 3.4.2.) or digested DNA from (Section 3.4.4.) from beneath the oil. Add the DNA to 40 µL of 0.1% SDS/10 mM EDTA and mix. Add 2 µL of this mixture to 2 µL of polyacrylamide gel loading dye and mix. The samples may be stored at –20°C for up to 1 wk before analyzing on a nondenaturing gel.

3.4.6. Preparation of Nondenaturing Gels

The DNA is analyzed on 0.3 mm × 40 cm × 30 cm, 6% polyacrylamide "nondenaturing" gels containing an *N,N'*-methylene bisacrylamide (*bis*) to acrylamide ratio of 1:20. The addition of 10% glycerol gives the best separation of normal and mutant DNA. However, it is possible that for certain mutations some variations of these conditions are necessary for detection (*see* Note 8).

Prepare the gel by mixing 27 mL of 40% acrylamide (bis:acrylamide 1:20), 18 mL of 10X TBE and 18 mL of glycerol. Adjust the volume to 180 mL with distilled water. Mix the gel gently on a magnetic stirrer for 15 min. Vigorous mixing should be avoided at this stage because undue aeration of the gel will prolong polymerization that, in turn, may result in excessive leakage of the gel. Before pouring the gel, add 130 µL of TEMED (*N,N,N',N'*-tetramethylethylenediamine) and 1.1 mL of freshly prepared 10% ammonium persulphate (APS) to the gel solution to catalyze polymerization. Store APS in a desiccator to prevent water absorption. After pouring the gel, insert the gel combs and leave it for 45 min to polymerize. After the gel has polymerized, cover the top with paper towels soaked in 1X TBE to prevent the wells from drying out.

3.4.7. Gel Electrophoresis

Leave the gel for at least 2 h at 4°C to ensure it cools sufficiently. One and a half liters of 1X TBE running buffer should also be left at 4°C. Electrophoresis at 4°C generally gives better separation of normal and mutant DNA *(8)* compared to room temperature. Air circulation systems, such as fans, create temperature gradients in the local environment that cause DNA samples to migrate faster on one side of the gel relative to the other. The position of the gel tank in the cold room is, therefore, critical to the accurate interpretation of gels. If the dye front does not run straight, it is essential that the gel tank is repositioned.

Prior to loading, denature the DNA samples at 95°C for 3 min. Rinse the gel wells using a syringe and needle in 1X TBE to remove residual polyacrylamide. Following denaturation, place the samples on ice immediately for 30 s to prevent renaturation then briefly microfuge and return to ice before loading them into the gel wells. Run at least six different samples for any one exon in adjacent wells so that any variation in the positions of the resultant bands can be seen clearly. An undenatured sample, which is not heated at 95°C, should also be analyzed to establish the position occupied by the double-stranded DNA. Electrophorese at 4°C for 4–6 h at 60 W in 1X TBE. The duration of electrophoresis is dependent on the length of the DNA fragments. Exons 7, 10, and 24 require a shorter run to preserve DNA <100 bp long and should be run until the xylene cyanol dye front is 5/8 of the way through the gel, which generally requires 4.5–5.5 h. For DNA fragments >110 bp, electrophorese the gels until the xylene cyanol lagging dye front has traversed 2/3 of the gel. Exons 10 and 24 require two runs on separate gels, a short one for fragments <100 bp and an additional run for 6 h to achieve adequate resolution of the larger fragments >200 bp.

Following electrophoresis, dry the gel in a vacuum gel dryer for 1–2 h. Fixation of SSCP gels is not required. Expose the gel to Kodak XAR-5 film for 12–72 h at –70°C without an intensifying screen that otherwise tends to blur the image.

Any samples that show differences in the final position of the bands on the gel (Fig. 1) should be sequenced as described herein.

There are several polymorphisms (Table 2) in the RB1 gene which will be detected using SSCP. The presence of a repeated pattern of bands in several DNA samples on SSCP gels may suggest a polymorphism. At least one of the samples showing such a pattern should be sequenced to confirm the presence of a polymorphism.

3.5. Sequencing of Biotin-Labeled Affinity Purified DNA

Once a bandshift is observed on an SSCP gel, the DNA should be sequenced to confirm and identify the mutation. There are several ways of sequencing directly from DNA produced using the PCR. Essential to the success of any direct sequencing protocol is the preparation of single-stranded DNA. One of the simplest and most reliable methods is to use the biotin/streptavidin magnetic bead procedure. In the protocol described in the following, one of the primers used to amplify the DNA template for sequencing is biotinylated. Streptavidin-coated magnetic beads to which biotin binds with a strong affinity are used to capture the biotinylated DNA. The nonbiotinylated strands are removed by denaturing the double-stranded DNA using sodium hydroxide and the DNA is ethanol precipitated. Thus, this procedure yields two relatively

Table 2
RB1 Polymorphisms

Exon	Location	Polymorphism	Ref.
4	23 bp in 3' intron	G or A	*15*
9	108 bp in 3' intron	9 or 10 T	Yandell[a]
10	58 bp in 3' intron	G or A	Yandell[a]
15	14 bp in 5' intron	A or T	Yandell[a]
26	10 bp in 5' intron	T or A	*16*

[a] Personal communication.

pure populations of single-stranded DNA that can be used as sequencing templates to confirm the mutation on both DNA strands. The principle is shown in the following (Fig. 2).

3.5.1. PCR Amplification

Amplify the relevant exon using PCR, as described in Section 3.3., using one primer (from Table 1) that has a biotin moiety attached during DNA synthesis at the 5' end (*see* Note 6).

Prepare the PCR reaction mixture on ice, as described in Section 3.3. except for the following modification. It is neccessary to reduce the amount of primers in the reaction to 5–15 pm to avoid saturating the streptavidin-coated beads with excess primer in preference to full-length PCR amplification products. The amount of primer required will vary from 5–15 pm and may need to be optimized if the intensity of the sequencing ladder is poor.

3.5.2. Purification of Single-Stranded DNA

1. Remove the supernatant from a 30-µL aliquot of resuspended magnetic streptavidin-coated beads. A magnetic rack is available from manufacturers of magnetic beads to immobilize the beads, allowing removal of supernatant.
2. Wash the beads twice with 100 µL of STE.
3. Remove the excess mineral oil from the amplified PCR product. Add the DNA to the washed beads and gently resuspend.
4. Adsorb the DNA to the beads for 5 min in a 28°C waterbath with occasional gentle mixing.
5. Following adsorption of the DNA to the beads, place the tube in the magnetic rack for 30 s and remove the supernatant (containing excess, unbound DNA) with a pipet.
6. Remove the tube from the magnet and resuspend the beads in freshly prepared 0.15*M* NaOH. Leave for 5 min to denature the double-stranded DNA.
7. Place the tube in the magnet for 30 s, remove the supernatant that contains the nonbiotinylated DNA and set aside.

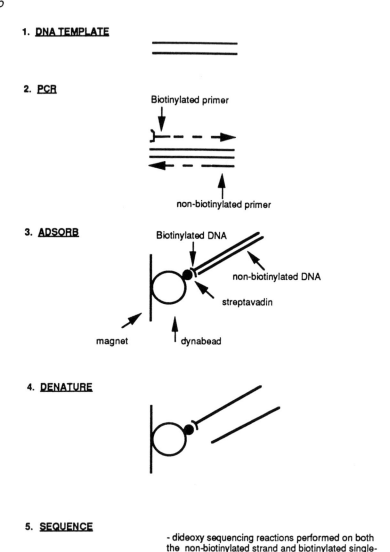

1. DNA TEMPLATE

2. PCR

Biotinylated primer

non-biotinylated primer

3. ADSORB

Biotinylated DNA

non-biotinylated DNA

streptavadin

magnet   dynabead

4. DENATURE

5. SEQUENCE

- dideoxy sequencing reactions performed on both
the non-biotinylated strand and biotinylated single-
stranded DNA

Fig. 2. Sequencing using magnetic streptavidin-coated beads (*see text* for details).

8. Wash the beads, with the biotinylated strand attached, in 100 μL of STE, followed by distilled deionized water and finally, resuspend in 5 μL of water.

   The immobilized biotinylated DNA can be sequenced while still bound to the
beads. The nonbiotinylated strand can be eluted and sequenced following ethanol
precipitation.

9. Precipitate the nonbiotinylated strands eluted in step 7 by adding 10 μL of 3M
sodium acetate, pH 5.2 and 250 μL of 100% ethanol and leave overnight at −70°C.

Table 3
Conditions for sequencing gels

Length from 3' end of primer	Polyacrylamide concentration	Time of electrophoresis, h
10–200 bp	6%	2
65–300 bp	6%	4
Up to 320 bp	4%	3

10. Recover the nonbiotinylated DNA by centrifugation at 12,000g in a microfuge for 20 min, wash the pellet in 75% ethanol, and resuspend in 5 μL of water.
11. Sequence the biotinylated and nonbiotinylated DNA using a dideoxy sequencing kit.

3.5.3. Sequencing

Any commercially available dideoxy sequencing kit should be suitable to use for sequencing. Adhere to the manufacturer's instructions, making sure to observe the following:

1. In order to ensure that extension from the primer during the labeling step (when dideoxy nucleotides are not present) is minimal, dilute the labelling mix 1:15 to allow the sequence close to the primer to be read.
2. For exon 17, use the 7-deaza-dGTP analog that forms weaker bonds with dCTP in place of dGTP. This will improve the quality of the sequencing for this exon.
3. Use either 4 or 6% polyacrylamide (0.3–0.6 mm) thick wedge gels for analyzing the products of sequencing reactions depending on the length of the sequence to be resolved on the sequencing gel (*see* Table 3).

3.5.4. Preparation of Sequencing Gels

1. Prepare 4 or 6% denaturing polyacrylamide gels (6 or 4% polyacrylamide, 7M urea). For 6% gels, combine 27 mL of 40% acrylamide (containing 1:20 *bis* acrylamide:acrylamide), 75.6 g of urea, 18 mL of 10X TBE pH 8.3, and water to 180 mL. For 4% gels, use 18 mL of 40% acrylamide. Dissolve the urea by gently heating the mixture. Pour a wedge gel (0.2–1.0 mm thick).
2. Flush the wells with 1X TBE using a needle and syringe before loading the samples onto the gel.
3. Denature the DNA samples at 95°C for 3 min before loading on the sequencing gel.
4. Electrophorese the gels at room temperature in 1X TBE buffer. The time of electrophoresis will depend on the length of the sequence to be read (*see* Table 3). It is also possible to do both a 2- and a 4-h run on the same gel by staggering the loading times.
5. Following electrophoresis fix the gel in a 10% methanol/10% acetic acid bath for 45 min.
6. Dry the gel in a vacuum dryer and expose to XAR-5 (Kodak, Rochester, NY) film overnight.

4. Notes

1. Inhibitors present in blood, such as hemoglobin, reduce the yield of product in the PCR reaction. A volume of 2 μL of blood is usually optimal. Using less blood decreases the yield of DNA because there is insufficient template present in the reaction. The proportion of inhibitors in the blood sample may vary between individuals and if a poor yield results, aliquots of blood ranging between 0.5 and 10 μL should be used to obtain the optimal yield of DNA.

2. The primers and conditions listed in Table 1 were optimized for a water-cooled thermocycler using a heating and cooling rate of 48°C/min, but should be suitable for any thermocycler.

3. Oligonucleotide primers are synthesized on a phosphoramidite column. Store the primers as a precipitate in 80% ethanol at −70°C until required, at which stage they should be spun in a microfuge for 10 min. Remove the supernatant and resuspend the pellet in H_2O or TE at a concentration of 0.5 mM.

4. It is necessary to store the dNTP mix in small aliquots so that they are not repeatedly thawed and frozen, otherwise, amplification soon deteriorates.

5. In order to reduce secondary structure, add 5 μL of dimethylsulfoxide to the reaction when exon 1 or the promoter region, which both have a high guanine and cytosine content, are amplified. Otherwise, aberrant PCR amplification products may be obtained.

6. The oligonucleotide primers used for SSCP can be biotinylated during synthesis if required for sequencing by the biotin/streptavidin magnetic bead method (*see* Section 3.5.1.). Biotinylation of oligonucleotide primers used for SSCP will not interfere with the detection of mutations by SSCP *(8)*.

7. If whole blood is used, prepare the sample as described in Section 3.2. If purified DNA is used, proceed to step 2 (Section 3.3.).

8. Studies of RB1 mutations in Rb tumors have demonstrated that 60% are point mutations, 30% are deletions (<50 bp), and 10% are insertions or complex mutations *(8,10)*. Similar results are now emerging from studies of mutations in lymphocytes from individuals with Rb *(17)*. RB1 mutations frequently generate premature stop codons *(10)*. Premature stop codons can arise as a result of frameshift mutations created by insertions or deletions or can be owing to point mutations. Arginine CGA codons in RB1 are frequently sites of CpG → TpG mutations creating TGA stop codons *(10,17)*.

    SSCP analysis will detect approx 70–75% of mutations in RB1 (Cowell, personal communication). The reason that mutations are not detected in all cases using SSCP is presumably because it is not 100% sensitive and may miss some mutations. Analysis at 4°C improves the sensitivity of SSCP significantly *(8)*. However, it is possible that for some mutations other conditions will be optimal and a second round of SSCP using different condition may be advisable. For instance, analysis of mutations at 4°C in gels lacking glycerol may be better for some mutations with less stable secondary structure.

    Problems may arise because SSCP may not detect large rearrangements or deletions. DNA in which mutations are not detected may require rescreening using Southern blotting. It would be advisable in a mutation screening program, however, to perform Southern blotting and cytogenetic analysis in those cases where a mutation was not detected by SSCP. In addition, it may be necessary to sequence every exon in those few cases when a mutation is not identified using SSCP.

Care must be taken in the interpretation of RB1 mutations. Most RB1 mutations will generate premature stop codons and there is evidence that missense mutations may be associated with a milder expression of the RB1 phenotype *(9,18)*. In addition, it is possible that rare polymorphisms occasionally may be detected.

References

1. Friend, S. H., Bernards, R., Rogelj, S, Weinberg, R. A, Rapaport, J. M., Albert, D. M., and Dryja, T. P. (1986) A human DNA segment with properties of the gene that predisposes to retinoblastoma and osteosarcoma. *Nature* **323,** 643–646.
2. Onadim, Z., Mitchell, C. D., Rutland, P. C., Buckle, B. G., Jay, M., Hungerford, J. L., Harper, K., and Cowell, J. K. (1990) Application of intragenic DNA probes in prenatal screening for retinoblastoma gene carriers in the United Kingdom. *Arch. Dis. Child* **65,** 651–656.
3. Wiggs, J., Nordenskjeld, M., Yandell, D., Rapaport, J., Grondin, V., Janson, M., Werelius, B., Petersen, R., Craft, A., Riedel, K., Lieberfarb, R., Walton, D., Wilson, W., and Dryja, T. P (1988) Prediction of the risk of hereditary retinoblastoma using DNA polymorphisms within the retinoblastoma gene. *N. Engl. J. Med.* **318,** 151–157.
4. Draper, G. J., Sanders, B. M., Brownbill, P. A., and Hawkins, M. M. (1992) Patterns of risk of hereditary retinoblastoma and applications to genetic counselling. *Br. J. Cancer* **66,** 211–219.
5. Orita, M., Suzuki, Y., Sekiya, T., and Hayashi, K. (1989) Rapid and sensitive detection of point mutations and DNA polymorphisms using the polymerase chain reaction. *Genomics* **5,** 874–879.
6. McGee, T. L., Yandell, D. W., and Dryja, T. P. (1989) Structure and partial genomic sequence of the human retinoblastoma susceptibility gene. *Gene* **80,** 119–128.
7. Dunn, J. M., Phillips, R. A, Zhu, X., Becker, A., and Gallie, B. L. (1989) Mutations in the RB1 gene and their effects on transcription. *Mol. Cell Biol.* **9,** 4596–4604.
8. Hogg, A. (1993). PhD thesis, University of London.
9. Kratzke, R. A., Otterson, G. A., Hogg, A., Coxon, A. B., Geradts, J., Cowell, J. K., and Kaye, F. J. (1994). Partial inactivation of the RB product in a family with incomplete penetrance of familial retinoblastoma and benign retinal tumors. *Oncogene* **9,** 1321–1326.
10. Hogg, A., Bia, B., Onadim, Z., and Cowell, J. K. (1993) Molecular mechanisms of oncogenic mutations in tumours from patients with bilateral and unilateral retinoblastoma. *PNAS* **90,** 7351–7355.

11. Cheng, J. and Maquat, L. E. (1993) Nonsense codons can reduce the abundance of nuclear mRNA without affecting the abundance of pre-mRNA or the half-life of cytoplasmic mRNA. *Mol. Cell Biol.* **13,** 1892–1902.

12. Urlaub, G., Mitchell, P. J., Ciudad, C. J., and Chasin, L. A. (1989) Nonsense mutations in the dihydrofolate reductase gene affect RNA processing. *Mol. Cell Biol.* **9,** 2868–2880.

13. Saiki, R. K., Gelfand, D. H., Stoffel, S., Scharf, S. J., Highuchi, R., Horn, G. T., Mullis, K. B., and Erlich, H. A. (1988) Primer-directed enzymatic amplification of DNA with a thermostable DNA polymerase. *Science* **239,** 487–491.

14. Hogg, A., Onadim, Z., Baird, P. N., and Cowell, J. K. (1992) Detection of heterozygous mutations in the RB1 gene in retinoblastoma patients using single-strand conformation polymorphism analysis and polymerase chain reaction sequencing. *Oncogene* **7,** 1445–1451.

15. Blanquet, V., Turleau, C., Goossens, M., and Besmond, C. (1992). A new G to T polymorphism in the retinoblastoma gene RB1 detected by DGGE. *NAR* **20,** 1432.

16. Yandell, D. W. and Dryja, T. P. (1989) Detection of DNA sequence polymorphisms by enzymatic amplification and direct genomic sequencing. *Am. J. Hum. Genet.* **45,** 547–555.

17. Cowell, J. K., Smith, T., and Bia, B. Frequent constitutional C $\rightarrow$ T mutations in CGA-arginine codons in the RB1 gene produce premature stop codons in patients with bilateral (hereditary) retinoblastoma, in press.

18. Onadim, Z., Hogg, A., Baird, P. N., and Cowell, J. K. (1992) Oncogenic point mutations in exon 20 of the RB1 gene in families showing incomplete penetrance and mild expression of the retinoblastoma phenotype. *PNAS* **89,** 6177–6181.

11

Mutational Analysis of the Wilms' Tumor (WT1) Gene

Linda King-Underwood and Kathy Pritchard-Jones

1. Introduction

Mutations of the Wilms' tumor (WT1) gene have been shown to underlie a proportion of cases of Wilms' tumor, an embryonal kidney cancer occurring mainly in childhood. The WT1 gene comprises ten exons spanning approx 50 kb of genomic DNA. The messenger RNA is approx 3 kb in length and encodes a zinc finger protein. The four zinc fingers, which lie at the C-terminal end of the protein, are encoded by separate exons 7–10. The 5' end of the gene is extremely GC-rich, with areas approaching a 70% GC content. This makes this region difficult to amplify in polymerase chain reactions.

Mutational analysis of the WT1 gene has been undertaken at both the DNA *(1–9)* and RNA level *(10,11)*. Most workers have used the single-stranded conformational polymorphism (SSCP) technique *(2–11)*, a few have used the mismatched-chemical cleavage technique *(1)*. Comparative studies have shown nearly equal sensitivity of these two techniques and of denaturing gradient gel electrophoresis (DGGE) in p53 mutational analysis *(12)*. An exon-by-exon approach has become the most commonly used for analysis of the WT1 gene coding region and splice donor and acceptor sites. One worker has attempted to speed up the process by using SSCP analysis of reverse transcribed RNA *(10,11)*. This generates large PCR products, of the order of 600 bp, which need to be digested with restriction enzymes down to a suitable length for optimal SSCP analysis. However, incomplete digestion of the PCR product may produce extra bands which falsely suggest the presence of mutation. This RNA-based approach does have the advantage that it will detect small deletions of entire exons and intronic mutations affecting splicing. Table 1 lists the primer sets used for WT1 gene mutational analysis in our laboratory (*see* Note 1). Many of these primer sequences were first chosen by other workers, as indicated.

From: *Methods in Molecular Medicine, Molecular Diagnosis of Cancer*
Edited by: F. E. Cotter Humana Press Inc., Totowa, NJ

Table 1
Primer Sequences and PCR Conditions for Amplification of Exons 1–10 of the WT1 Gene

Exon	Primer name	Ref.	Primer sequence 5' to 3'	Final Mg^{2+}, mM	Annealing temp., °C	Product size, bp
1	B1 or	(11)	AGCAGTGCCTGAGCGCCTT	1.5^a	65	251
	C550		CCGCCTCACTCCTTCATCA	1.5^a	65	309
	JR1		TCCTAGAGCGGGAGAGTCCCTG			
2	C147		AAGCTTGCGAGAGCACCGCTG	1.0^a	59	231
	3 × 2	(7)	AGAGGAGGATAGCACGGAAG			
3	C149		GGCTCAGGATCTCGTGTCTC	1.0^a	60	271
	C150		CCAAGTCCGCCGGCTCATG			
4	C486		AAACAGTTGTGTATTATTTTGTGG	1.5	55	225
	C152		ACTTTCTTCATAAGTTCTAAGCAC			
5	C153		CAGATCCATGCATGCTCCATTC	1.0	55	176
	C154		CTCTTGCATTGCCCCAGGTG			
6	C178		AAGCTTCACTGACCCTTTTCCCTTC	2.0	55	231
	C177		GAATTCCAAAGAGTCCATCAGTAAGG			
7	C155		GACCTACGTGAATGATCACATG	1.5	50	349
	945	(1)	ACAACACCTGGATCAAGACCT			
8	C323		CCTTTAATGAGATCCCCTTTTCC	1.5	55	191
	3 × 8	(7)	AGGGAACACAGCTCGCAGCAATGAG			
9	5 × 9	(7)	TAGGGCCGAGGCTAGACCTTCTCTG	1.5	60	204
	3 × 9	(7)	ATCCCTCTCATCACAATTTCATTCC			
10	5 × 10	(7)	GTTGCAAGTGTCTCTGACTGG	2.0	59	235
	B4	(9)	GGAGTGGAGAGTCAGACTTG			

Primers are listed in pairs with 5' (sense) first, followed by the 3' (antisense).
^{a}These primer pairs required the addition of 1% formamide to the reaction mixture. Primer sequence prefixed C were selected at the MRC Human Genetics Unit, Edinburgh.

2. Materials

Stock solution should be aliquoted into volumes suitable for performing 50–100 PCR reactions, so that each aliquot is only in use for a few days. The "master mix" for the PCR reaction should be set up either before the DNAs to be analyzed are handled or after a change of gloves (*see* Note 2).

1. Plasticware: Plasticware (i.e., microfuge tubes and tips) is either purchased as sterile items or autoclaved. Plugged tips are used throughout.
2. Water: Sterile distilled or deionized water is used and kept in aliquots specifically for PCR to avoid contamination.
3. 10X PCR buffer: 500 m*M* KCl (1*M* autoclaved stock), 100 m*M* Tris-HCl, pH 8.3 (1*M* autoclaved stock), 10–20 m*M* MgCl$_2$ (1*M* autoclaved stock), and 0.01% gelatin (1 mg/1 mL filter sterilized stock). Make up in sterile distilled water and store at –20°C in small aliquots.
4. 50X dNTPs for standard PCR: 10 m*M* each of dATP, dCTP, dGTP, and dTTP diluted with sterile distilled water from commercially available 100 m*M* solutions. Store at –20°C in small aliquots.
5. 50X dNTPs for SSCP: 10 m*M* each dATP, dGTP and dTTP; 1 m*M* dCTP diluted with sterile distilled water from commercially available 100 m*M* solutions. Store at –20°C in small aliquots.
6. Oligonucleotide primers: Dilute to 25 µ*M* and store in small aliquots at –20°C.
7. Formamide dye (stop solution): 95% formamide, 20 m*M* EDTA, and 0.05% each of bromophenol blue and xylene cyanol FF. Store at –20°C in small aliquots.
8. 40% acrylamide: bisacrylamide solution, 19:1. This can be purchased from many suppliers. Store at 4°C.
9. 10X TBE: 108 g Tris-base, 55 g boric acid, and 40 mL of 0.5*M* EDTA. Make up to 1 L and autoclave. Store at room temperature.
10. Ammonium persulfate 10%: One gram of ammonium persulfate is dissolved in 10 mL distilled water. This should be made fresh each time or stored at –20°C.
11. TEMED: *N'* Tetramethylethylenediamine.
12. Glycerol
13. α^{32}P dCTP.

3. Methods

3.1. SSCP

For convenience, PCRs are usually carried out overnight and run on gels during the next day. Up to 40 samples, plus controls, can be run on one gel. Polyacrylamide gels are poured and allowed to cool to 4°C overnight.

3.1.1. Genomic DNA PCR

1. 50–100 ng of genomic DNA are diluted to 5 µL with water in 0.5-mL microfuge tubes and placed at 4°C until required.
2. The remaining ingredients are mixed at room temperature in a 1.5-mL screw-cap microfuge tube as follows, scaling up the volumes for the number of samples and adding the required amount of water first. The mix per sample is: 2.5 µL 10X

PCR buffer, 0.5 μL 50X dNTP mix for SSCP, 0.5 μL each of the two primers, 0.1 μL (0.1 μCi) α³²P dCTP, 0.5 U *Taq* polymerase, and water to 20 μL.

3. Flick the tube and centrifuge to collect all the liquid at the bottom. To the diluted DNA (5 μL) add 20 μL of reaction mix (total reaction volume 25 μL). A small volume of mineral oil (one drop) is then added to stop evaporation, and the tubes are immediately transferred to the PCR heating block.

4. Amplification is carried out as follows using the annealing temperatures shown in Table 1 (*see* Note 3):
   a. 1st cycle: 94°C for 4 min, annealing temperature for 1 min, and 72°C for 2 min.
   b. 2nd to 35th cycle: 94°C for 30 s, annealing temperature for 1 min, and 72°C for 1 min.
   c. Final cycle: 72°C for 5 min.

3.1.2. Acrylamide Gel Electrophoresis

1. A 6% acrylamide, 10% glycerol gel is prepared. The standard sequencing gel format is used with 0.4-mm spacers and a 48-well sharkstooth comb. For 80-mL of gel solution the following ingredients are mixed: 52 mL water, 8 mL 10X TBE, 8 mL glycerol, and 12 mL 40% acrylamide stock. Forty microliters of TEMED and 300 μL of 10% ammonium persulfate is added immediately before pouring the gel. Once it is fully polymerized, the gel is put at 4°C overnight, along with the required amount of 1X TBE for the sequencing gel electrophoresis tank.

2. Following amplification, the tubes are briefly centrifuged. Some 2–4 μL from each reaction are added to 8 μL of formamide dye in a 0.5-mL tube and heat-denatured at 95°C for 3 min. A duplicate tube of one or two samples is not heated, to serve as a double-stranded control. Two-and-one-half microliters of each sample are loaded onto the gel and electrophoresed at 40W for 5–6 h at 4°C.

3. At the end of the run, transfer the gel to filter paper and dry using an 80°C gel drier. Expose the dried gel to X-ray film for 1–5 d at room temperature, or for shorter times at –70°C with intensifying screens. Some examples of SSCP gels are shown in Fig. 1. (*see* Notes 4–7).

3.2. Sequencing of Mutations

Samples with altered band patterns are checked by direct sequencing of purified PCR products, using the PCR primers or internal primers where required. Set up 2 × 50 μL PCR reactions for each sample, using the same recipe as for the SSCP PCRs, but using standard 50 × dNTPs and omitting the radiolabeled dCTP. The PCR program remains the same as for SSCP. Cut the PCR products out of low melting-point agarose gels and purify using Wizard PCR Preps (Promega) (*see* Note 8). Sequencing is carried out using Sequenase (Amersham) in a method optimized for double-stranded PCR products *(13)* (*see* Note 9). Alternatively, the purified PCR products can be subcloned into plasmid or bacteriophage vectors designed for that purpose, although many clones have to be sequenced for each sample to eliminate errors caused by *Taq* polymerase during the amplification process. Some examples of sequencing results are shown in Fig. 2.

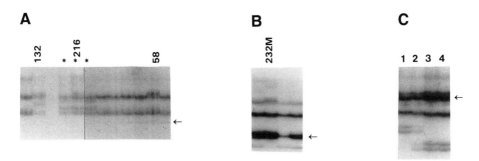

Fig. 1. SSCP of exons 7, 8, and 9 of WT1. Arrows mark the position at which the double-stranded PCR products migrated. Unmarked lanes are samples with normal sequence. Numbered lanes are samples found to contain mutations. **(A)** Exon 7. *, samples heterozygous for the A/G polymorphism at the beginning of the exon. **(B)** Exon 9. **(C)** Exon 8. Three different band patterns can be seen but all the samples had wild-type sequence.

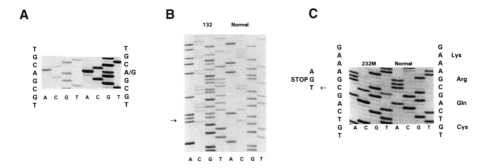

Fig. 2. Sequencing of samples with altered SSCP bands. **(A)** The 5' end of exon 7 showing an individual homozygous A/A (left) and one heterozygous A/G (right). **(B)** The 5' end of exon 7 showing sample 132, which has a heterozygous 5-bp insertion after codon 300. The altered sequence is superimposed on the sequence of the normal allele, starting at the arrow. **(C)** Part of exon 9 showing a heterozygous C to T point mutation in sample 232M, which changes Arginine[390] CGA to a STOP codon TGA.

4. Notes

1. The primer sequences shown in Table 1 are used mainly because they were available in the laboratory and in general gave a suitably sized product. However, we have not compared several different primer pairs for each exon so these are not necessarily the optimal combinations for SSCP. Some of the PCR products cover intron sequences containing polymorphisms, which, while they are useful posi-

tive controls for the SSCP, may complicate the band patterns. The PCR product for exon 3 contains two polymorphisms. The first is a C to T change in the 5' intron 21 bp downstream of primer C149 and the second is a G to A change 16 bp downstream from the end of the exon sequence. The 3' primer for this exon could be replaced by that used by Gessler et al. *(2)*. There is a T to G polymorphism in the exon 7 product, 5 bp upstream of primer 945. Gessler et al. *(2)* use a different primer, which could be substituted for 945 and would avoid this polymorphism. Two different 5' primers are shown for exon 1. Exon 1 is very GC rich and thus difficult to amplify. Either set of primers works well, but both only cover the 3' end of the exon.

2. All work involving amplication by the polymerase chain reaction must be exercised with extreme caution to prevent contamination of stock solutions. Measures should include having a dedicated set of pipets for PCR set-up work and the use of plugged pipet tips. Mixing of solutions by pipeting up and down should be avoided. Stock solutions should be made in bulk using sterile distilled water taken from a laboratory where there is no plasmid work with the same gene.

3. These conditions are for a Hybaid Omnigene thermal cycler with a tube thermistor. Times may need to be adjusted for other manufacturers' machines, particularly if they use block or simulated tube temperature control.

4. The decision as to whether an individual sample shows an altered banding pattern can sometimes be difficult. If a subtle blurring of the band is seen, then rerunning of the PCR products for a much longer electrophoresis time may resolve an altered band. When a consistently altered band is seen in several unrelated samples, this usually represents either a polymorphism or lack of mutation that can be detected on direct sequencing. Sometimes the altered band pattern is unexplained.

5. Optimization of the SSCP conditions in terms of gel glycerol content, TBE composition, and electrophoresis temperature and speed has to be performed with a known mutant for each exon as a positive control. If no naturally occurring mutants are available, then they can be created by cloning PCR products for that particular exon and sequencing a sufficient number (usually 10–20) to detect a point mutation introduced by the *Taq* polymerase.

6. Some of the exons also contain silent base changes in the coding sequence. Exon 1 has a C to T change at the third base of Asparagine 130 and exon 7 has an A to G change at the third base of Arginine 301 (Figs. 1 and 2).

7. Figure 1C shows the band patterns seen for exon 8. Similar bands were seen under different gel-running conditions, always in the same samples. Samples with all three different patterns have been sequenced several times but all are completely normal. No explanation for the altered bands has been suggested so far.

8. A variety of other methods are available for purifying PCR products.

9. Many sequencing methods have been published and may be equally as good (*see also* protocol in Chapter 12 [Booth]).

References

1. Little, M. H., Prosser, J., Condie, A., Smith, P. J., Van Heyningen, V., and Hastie, N. D. (1992) Zinc finger point mutations within the WT1 gene in Wilms' tumor patients. *Proc. Natl. Acad. Sci. USA* **89,** 4791–4795.
2. Gessler, M., Knig, A., Arden, K., Grundy, P., Orkin, S., Sallan, S., Peters, C., Ruyle, S., Mandell, J., Li, F., Cavenee, W., and Bruns, G. (1994) Infrequent mutation of the WT1 gene in 77 Wilms' tumours. *Hum. Mutat.* **3,** 212–222.
3. Park, S., Bernard, A., Bove, K. E., Sens, D. A., Hazen-Martin, D. J., Garvin, J. A., and Haber, D. A. (1993) Activation of WT1 in nephrogenic rests, genetic precursors to Wilms' tumour. *Nat. Genet.* **5,** 363–367.
4. Park, S., Schyalling, M., Bernard A., Maheswaren, S., Shipley, G. C., Roberts, D., Fletcher, J., Shipman, R., Rheinwald, J., Demetri, G., Griffin, J., Minden, M., Housman, D., and Haber, D. (1993) The Wilms' tumour gene WT1 is expressed in murine mesoderm-derived tissues and mutated in a human mesothelioma. *Nat. Genet.* **4,** 415–419.
5. Coppes, M. J., Van Liefers, G., Paul, P., Heger, H., and Williams, B. R. G. (1993) Homozygous somatic WT1 point mutations in sporadic unilateral Wilms' tumour. *Proc. Natl. Acad. Sci. USA* **90,** 1416–1419.
6. Varanasi, R., Bardeesy, N., Ghahremani, M., Petruzzi, M.-J., Nowak, N., Adam, M. A., Cundy, P., Shows, T. B., and Pelletier, J. (1994) Fine structure analysis of the WT1 gene in sporadic Wilms' tumors. *Proc. Natl. Acad. Sci. USA* **91,** 3554–3558.
7. Baird, P. N., Groves, N., Haber, D. A., Houseman, D. E., and Cowell, J. K. (1992) Identification of mutations in the WT1 gene in tumours from patients with the WAGR syndrome. *Oncogene* **7,** 2141–2149.
8. Huff, V., Jaffe, N., Saunders, G. F., Strong, L. C., Villalba, F., and Ruteshouser, E. C. (1995) WT1 exon 1 deletion/insertion mutations in Wilms' tumor patients, associated with di- and trinucleotide repeats and deletion hotspot consensus sequences. *Am. J. Hum. Genet.* **56,** 84–90.
9. Pritchard-Jones, K., Renshaw, J., and King-Underwood, L. (1994) The Wilms' tumour (WT1) gene is mutated in a secondary leukaemia in a WAGR patient. *Hum. Mol. Genet.* **3,** 1633–1637.
10. Brown, K. W., Wilmore, H. P., Watson, J. E., Mott, M. G., BelTy, J., and Maitland, N. J. (1993) Low frequency of mutations in the WT1 coding region in Wilms' tumor. *Genes, Chromosomes and Cancer* **8,** 74–79.
11. Brown, K. W., Watson, J. L, Poirier, J., Mott, M. G., Berry, P. J., and Maitland, N. J. (1992) Inactivation of the remaining allele of the WT1 gene in a Wilms' tumour from a WAGR patient. *Oncogene* **7,** 763–768.
12. Condie, A., Eeles, R. A., Boresen, A. L, Coles, C. and Cooper C. S. (1993) Deletion of point mutations in the p53 gene, comparison of SSCP, CDGE, and HOT. *Hum. Mutat.* **2,** 58–66.
13. King-Underwood, L., Renshaw, J., and Pritchard-Jones, K. (1996) Mutations in the Wilms' tumour gene WT1 in leukaemias. *Blood* **87,** 2171–2179.

III

GENERAL TECHNIQUES
FOR CANCER ANALYSIS

12

Single-Strand Conformation Polymorphism Mutation Analysis of the p53 Gene

Mark J. Booth

1. Introduction

Single-strand conformation polymorphism (SSCP) is a rapid and convenient procedure by which differences in the base composition of short DNA strands may be detected *(1,2)*. A useful application of this is in the comparison of polymerase chain reaction (PCR) generated products from gene coding sequences of unknown or patient material with a known wild-type standard; where any deviation of the banding pattern produced by the former from that produced by the latter indicates a possible mutation within the sequence of that product.

The principle of this technique is shown in summary in Fig. 1. Through a modified PCR, radiolabeled products of the unknown and wild-type sequence are produced. These strands are then heat denatured and subsequently separated by electrophoresis on a nondenaturing polyacrylamide gel. Under these conditions the single-stranded DNA will form a unique secondary structure owing to intra-strand hydrogen-bonds and base-stacking, wholly dependent on the base composition. Separation during electrophoresis is then determined solely by the different migration rates of the structures so formed. Autoradiographic detection of the banding pattern produced by each PCR product indicates any migrational differences of the unknown from the wild-type and a need to then sequence that product for conformation and clarification of the mutation present.

The advantages of SSCP over other techniques of mutational analysis (such as RNase protection, chemical cleavage mismatch, or denaturing gradient gel electrophoreses) is its relative simplicity and speed with which a large number of samples may be screened simultaneously. Under suitable conditions this technique is capable of detecting over 90% of mutations occurring within any sequence; as little as 1 nucleotide change causing an easily identifiable band shift.

From: *Methods in Molecular Medicine, Molecular Diagnosis of Cancer*
Edited by: F. E. Cotter Humana Press Inc., Totowa, NJ

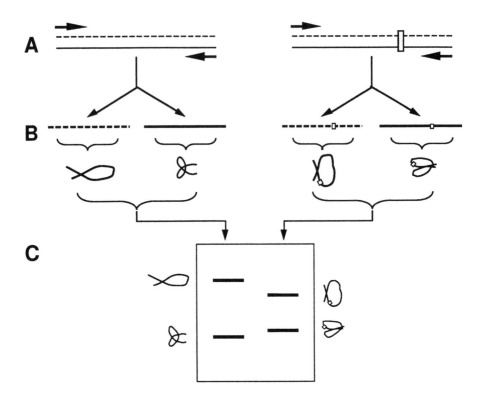

Fig. 1. Schematic of SSCP procedure for mutational analysis: **(A)** Modified PCR creates radiolabeled product from known normal and unknown mutated (□) template. **(B)** Heat denaturation and snap-cooling reduces DNA to single strands and allows unique intrastrand secondary structure to form. **(C)** Nondenaturing PAGE allows separation of the strands detectable by autoradiography. Band shifts in the unknown indicate possible presence of mutation.

p53 is already well characterized as one of the most frequently altered genes *(3)*, up to 60–70% within a diverse variety of malignancies *(4)*. Although spanning over 20 kb much is repetitive and generally it is acknowledged that the most frequently observed mutations are point mutations within the highly conserved regions spanned by exons 5–9, with as many as 90% identified in exons 5, 7, and 8 *(5)*. SSCP then, provides an ideal technique for basic mutational analysis of this p53 "hotspot" region.

As with all protocols involving the use of radiolabelled ligands (particularly ^{32}P), especial care should be taken and all advised safety precautions strictly adhered to: i.e., a designated and isolated work area; at least 1 cm of perspex shielding between any isotope and the operator at all times.

Consideration of the PCR reaction is of significant importance for successful analysis by SSCP. A single, well-defined product is required and good primer design is therefore essential to limit any nonspecific priming. For suggested primers *see* Fig. 2. GC rich regions should be avoided as these tend to be areas of secondary structure, whereas areas of high AT content will reduce annealing temperatures and may therefore contribute to background products. Primers of 20–25 bps in length with a 45–55% GC content and avoiding primer end complementarity are usually satisfactory for SSCP requirements. Annealing within the intron, 30–50 bps away from the exon, allows the inclusion of splice site and branch point regions within the analysis. Suitable cycle temperatures and times will vary depending on the machine used, but it has been generally found that those listed have proven adequate with the primers suggested. Ramp rates should be at the maximum available and cycle number not excessive or reaction specificity may be reduced; 40 generally being a maximum.

PCR-SSCP analysis is limited in that it can only be used to differentiate a mutationally altered product from the normal if the DNA template population of the suspected mutant contains at least 10% mutated sequence. It may therefore be necessary in some cases to enrich for the suspected mutant DNA prior to analysis; such as flow sorting of a specific neoplastic component from a heterogeneous cell population where contaminating normal cells are in a greater than 90% majority *(5)*.

The final factor of prime importance in being able to determine whether a mutation is present or not is the content of the polyacrylamide gel and the conditions under which it is run. The suggested conditions for this protocol will allow 90% of mutations to be detected. However, it should be made aware that other sets of conditions for successful running and band shift determination are not only possible, but necessary if 100% of all possible mutations are to be identified. Suggested alternatives of gel/run permutations therefore have been made *(6)*.

2. Materials

1. 10X *Taq* polymerase reaction buffer: 500 mM KCl, 100 mM Tris-HCl, pH 9.0, 1.0% v/v Triton X-100, 1.5 mM MgCl$_2$.
2. Nucleotide mix: 2 mM dATP, 2 mM dGTP, 2 mM dTTP, 0.2 mM dCTP.
3. Primers: phosphoramidite synthesized, fully deprotected, and stored at 20 μM in TE (10 mM Tris-HCl, pH 7.5, 1 mM EDTA).
4. Template DNA: ~100 ng/μL in H$_2$O or TE.
5. Amplification dilution buffer: 0.1% w/v SDS, 10 mM EDTA.
6. Formamide loading buffer: 95% v/v formamide, 20 mM EDTA, 0.05% w/v bromophenol blue, 0.05% w/v xylene cyanol.
7. 5X TBE running buffer: 0.45M Tris-borate, 0.01M EDTA.

All reagents may be aliquoted and stored at –20°C, except TBE at RT.

Exon 5   (2832-3329)

agctcgctag tgggttgcag gaggtgctta cacatgtttg tttctttgct

gccgtgttcc agttgcttta tctgttcact tgtgccctga ctttcaactc

tgtctccttc ctcttcctac agtactcccc tgccctcaac aagatgtttt
                              126

gccaactggc caagacctgc cctgtgcagc tgtgggttga ttccacaccc

ccgcccggca cccgcgtccg cgccatggcc atctacaagc agtcacagca
    HpaII   NcoI

catgacggag gttgtgaggC GCtgccccca ccatgagcgc tgctcagata
                    175

gcgatggtga gcagctgggg ctggagagac gacagggctg gttgcccagg

gtcccaggc ctctgattcc tcactgattg ctcttaggtc tggcccc

Exon 7   (3888-4209)

tgggcgacag agcgagattc catctcaaaa aaaaaaaaaa aaggcctccc

ctgcttgcca caggtctccc caaggcgcac tggcctcatc ttgggcctgt

gttatctcct aggttggctc tgactgtacc accatccact acaactacat
              225   Rsal   248 249

gtgtaacagt tcctgcatgg gcGGCatgaa CCGGAGGccc atcctcacca
                          245   HpaII

tcatcacact ggaagactcc aggtcaggag ccacttgcca ccctgcacac

tggcctgctg tgccccagcc tctgcttgcc gctgacccct gggcccagct

cttaccgatt tcttccatac ta

Exon 8   (4362-4678)

tgggagtaga tggagcctgg tttttaaat gggacaggta ggacctgatt

tccttactgc ctcttgcttc tcttttccta tcctgagtag tggtaatcta
                                                    262

ctgggacgga acagctttga ggtgCGTgtt tgtgcctgtc ctgggagaga
    282   273

CCGGcgcaca gaggaagaga atctccgcaa gaaaggggag cctcaccacg
HpaII   MboI

agctgccccc agggagcact aagcgaggta agcaagcagg acaagaagcg

gtggaggaga ccaagggtgc agttatgcct cagattcact tttatcacct

ttccttgcct ctttcct

Fig. 2. Sequence data for exons 5, 7, and 8 (5'–3') with flanking intron boundaries for p53. Sequence in bold indicates exon sequence with the first codon in each is numbered. Hotspot mutation codons are denoted by uppercase and also labeled with codon number. ➤ denotes suggested SSCP PCR primers; — ➤ alternative primers; – – ➤ exon boundary sequencing primers; ☐ suggested restriction enzyme site.

3. Methods

3.1. PCR Labeling

1. For each sample prepare on ice in 0.5-mL microfuge tubes in the following order: 35 µL H_2O, 5 µL *Taq* polymerase 10X reaction buffer, 5 µL dNTP mix, 1 µL each primer, 1 µL template DNA, 100 µLs (~2 drops) mineral oil, 1 µL 1:10 dilution in H_2O of α-^{32}P dCTP 3000 Ci/mmol, 1 U *Taq* polymerase.

2. Pulse spin in microfuge and place in thermal cycler programmed to run:

	94°C	4 min	
Denaturation	94°C	45–60 s	
Annealing	55–58°C	30–60 s	} 30–40 cycles
Extension	72°C	1–2 min	
	72°C	10 min.	

3. Ten-microliter aliquots from each PCR reaction should be checked on a 1.8% agarose gel to ensure a single product of good quantity and the correct size has been generated. Samples may be subsequently stored at –20°C.

4. Optional PCR product digestion: Remove 15 µL PCR product and add approx 8 U of restriction enzyme. Digest 12–16 h at 37°C (or enzyme used optimal temperature). Check a 5-µL aliquot on 1.8% agarose for good digestion. Digestions may be subsequently stored at –20°C.

5. Dilute samples at some point prior to gel running: 5-µL sample (PCR product or digestion); 25–40 µL amplification dilution buffer. Mix and pulse in microfuge, may then be stored at –20°C.

3.2. SSCP Polyacrylamide Gel Electrophoresis (PAGE)

1. Pour 6% nondenaturing polyacrylamide gel. Suggested mix (for alternatives *see* Note 6): 27 mL 40% acrylamide (1:20 *bis*:acryl), 36 mL 5X TBE, 18 mL glycerol, 99 mL H_2O, final vol 180 mL. To catalyze polymerization add: 180 µL Temed, 130 µL fresh 25% w/v ammonium persulfate. Pour immediately.

2. Gels to be run at 4°C should be prechilled for at least 2 h along with sufficient 1X TBE running buffer (although overnight is better).

3. Prior to loading, gels should be run for 30 min, to achieve temperature stability.

4. For each sample to be run, in a fresh 0.5-mL microfuge tube add: 3 µL diluted sample, 3 µL formamide loading buffer. Two tubes should be prepared for the known nonmutated control sample.

5. Denature all samples except one of the nonmutated controls at 94°C for 3 min. Transfer to ice for 3 min, quickly pulse spin in microfuge, then put back onto ice.

6. Load 5 µL of each sample, one in each well, most importantly including both the denatured and nondenatured known nonmutated control samples.

7. Suggested running conditions for the above gel (for alternatives *see* Note 6): 4 h at 60 W constant power at 4°C ambient temperature.

8. Post-running, gels are blotted off onto 3MM cartridge paper and dried down under vacuum at 80°C for 30–60 min.

9. Subsequent autoradiographic exposure to Kodak X-OMAT film for 12–16 h, without screens at –70°C should give sufficient banding patterns for analysis and mutation-containing sample identification.

4. Notes

1. A control DNA template of known, nonmutated sequence must be included as well as any unknowns, and run as both denatured and nondenatured.

2. For multiple samples reaction mix may be prepared in bulk by adding $n + 1$ (where n is the number of samples) amounts of all reagents except template and mineral oil. This is then aliquoted into 0.5-mL microfuge tubes containing the template and mineral oil is then added.

3. Annealing temperatures and time at each step of the cycling should, for initial runs, be started high and short, respectively; decreasing and lengthening if no product is obtained. SSCP requirement is for a single, well-defined product and if this cannot be obtained by altering cycle temperature/times (especially for annealing) then 10% DMSO may be added to the reaction mix (in place a corresponding amount of the water). This may improve the specificity of the reaction and has been shown not to interfere with latter fragment migration on the polyacrylamide gel.

4. Alternative protocols suggest using end-labeled primers for labeling of PCR products, which could simplify the PCR protocol and reportedly cuts down on background on the polyacrylamide gel.

5. It has been noted generally that SSCP identification of band shifts on polyacrylamide gels is best determined when the DNA fragments involved are between 150–200 bp in length *(7)*. With fragments much above 250 bp, mutation detection begins to fall below 90%. For this reason it is advisable to digest lengthy fragments to more suitable sizes before PAGE. Although this will create a more complex banding pattern due to increased strand number, band shifts are likely to be more pronounced. For this reason suitable restriction enzyme cut-sites have been indicated on the sequence data (Fig. 2). Fragments produced should ideally be between 150–200 bp (as a decreased mutation detection below the 150 threshold has also been noted) and with a 30-bp difference between them to ensure their dissimilar migration on polyacrylamide. Note that the *Taq* buffer has proven adequate for the digestion reaction in this case.

6. The inclusion of glycerol in the gel acts as a mild denaturant aiding in the separation of bands by opening the secondary structure a little. However, this can retard the gel running and reduce distances between dsDNA and ssDNA. Compensating for this by running the gel at higher power can significantly increase gel temperature and disturb secondary structure best retained at low temperature. Low running power can result in more diffuse bands and make identification of closely migrating bands in the same sample difficult. The suggested gel/running conditions are a good compromise between speed and resolution. Suggested alternatives include:

Glycerol		Hours
+10%	30–60 W	4–6 h at 4°C
+10%	10–20 W	6–12 h at 4°C
+10%	300–500 W	12–16 h at 4°C
Without	10–30 V	4–8 h at RT
Without	300–500 V	12–16 h at RT

Polyacrylamide gel mix and subsequent running conditions listed refer to the Gibco-BRL (Gaithersburg, MD) Model S2 system routinely used where the gel dimensions are:

Height	×	Width	×	Thickness
400 mm		300 mm		0.4 mm

and sharks-tooth combs providing wells 10 mm wide were used.

7. It has been noted that gel porosity can affect band migration on the polyacrylamide gel; a decrease in the *bis*:acryl. ratio by as much as 1:100 possibly increasing band separation and shortening run time required.

8. A preference for well former combs rather than sharks-tooth has been noted as the latter may cause band curvature across the gel.

9. Gel tanks should be set up to run in positions free from drafts and temperature fluctuations as any variance across the gel can cause a pronounced uneven band migration across it and complicate detection of shifts. Screening the gel from air currents, especially those run at 4°C, has been found to be a good idea and easily accomplished by prodigious use of a large cardboard box placed over or around the tank.

10. The exact dilution of the sample in dilution buffer will depend on the amount of product produced and the strength and quality of the signal incorporated. Initially, 5 µL of sample in 30 µL of buffer would appear adequate. If signal or background produced is too strong then the dilution can be increased and if weak then reduced.

11. Wells/top of the gel should be washed well before loading using the running buffer in a 25–30-mL syringe. Lanes at the far edges of the gel should be avoided as these are more prone to distorted running. Use of duck-billed pipet tips was found to facilitate easier loading into the wells.

12. Post-running fixation of the gel is not required although any wrinkles caused by plate separation can be smoothed out in 10% methanol, 10% glacial acetic acid.

13. Banding patterns produced are likely to be more complex than at first would be expected. A single ssDNA species is likely to produce three to four bands owing to a number of different metastable secondary conformations that it can take; although more intense bands will indicate those most strongly favored. (*See* Fig. 3). As well as a dsDNA band, other aberrant bands can be caused by heteroduplex formations between normal and mutant strands if both are generated within the same sample and for this reason the running of denatured and nondenatured normal controls is vital.

    Although a rare occurrence, instances of migration changes of bands have been observed by SSCP analysis that could not be identified by subsequent sequence analysis.

    Note that the identification of a band of altered mobility is easier from a gel on which multiple samples have been run *(8,9)*.

14. Use of biotinylated sequencing primers for SSCP PCR can retard the mobility of the strands produced on the polyacrylamide gel but as shifts should be the same for both sample and control, a migratory property alteration owing to a mutation should still be identifiable.

15. The majority of mutations within p53 are seen as transitions at CpG dinucleotides; sites of spontaneous mutation due to deamination of 5-methylcytosine residues.

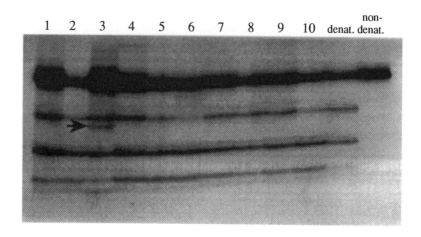

Fig. 3. Example of SSCP mutation analysis of p53, exon 8. 10 unknown samples are shown along with the denatured and nondenatured normal control. The migrational difference of the band in lane 3 is clearly evident and indicates that this sample should be sequenced for mutation conformation and clarification.

References

1. Orita, M., Iwahana, H., Kanazawa, H., Hayashi, K., and Sekiya, T. (1989a) Rapid and sensitive detection of point mutations and DNA polymorphism's using the polymerase chain reaction. *Proc. Natl. Acad. Sci. USA* **86,** 2766–2770.
2. Orita, M., Suzuki, Y., Sekiya, T., and Hayashi, K. (1989b) Detection of polymorphism's of human DNA by gel electrophoresis as single strand conformation polymorphism's. *Genomics* **5,** 874–879.
3. Levine, A. (1992) p53 tumour suppressor gene and product. *Cancer Surveys* **12,** 59–79.
4. Nigro, J., Baker, S., Preisinger, A., Jessup, J., Hostetter, R., Cleary, K., Bigner, S., Davidson N., Baylin, S., Devilee, P., Glover, T., Collins, F., Weston, A., Harris, C., and Vogelstein, B. (1989) Mutations in the p53 gene occur in diverse human tumour types. *Nature* **342,** 705.
5. Gupta, R. K., Patel, K., Bodmer, W. F., and Bodmer, J. G. (1992) Mutation of p53 in primary biopsy material and cell lines from Hodgkin disease. *Proc. Natl. Acad. Sci. USA* **90,** 2817–2821.
6. Spinardi, L., Mazars, R., and Theillet, C. (1991) Protocols for an improved detection of point mutations by SSCP. *Nucleic Acid Res.* **19(14),** 4009.
7. Sheffield, V. C., Beck, J. S., Kwitek, A. E., Sandstrom, D. W., and Stone, E. M. (1993) The sensitivity of single strand conformation polymorphism analysis for the detection of single base substitutions. *Genomics* **16,** 325–332.
8. Baldini, L., Fracchiolla, N. S., Cro, L. M., Trecca, D., Romitti, L., Polli, E., Maiolo, A. T., and Neri, A. (1994) Frequent p53 gene involvement in splenic B-cell leukemia/lymphomas of possible marginal zone origin. *Blood* **84(1),** 270–278.

9. Neri, A., Balcini, L., Trecca, D., Cro, E. P., and Maiolo, A. T. (1993) p53 gene mutations in multiple myeloma are associated with advanced forms of malignancy. *Blood* **81(1),** 128–135.

Further Reading

Maniatis, T., Fritsch, E. F., and Sambrook, J. (1982) *Molecular Cloning: A Laboratory Manual.* Cold Spring Harbor Laboratory Press, Cold Spring Harbor, NY.

Levine, A. J. (1992) *Tumour Suppressor Genes, The Cell Cycle and Cancer,* vol. 12, Cold Spring Harbor Laboratory Press, Cold Spring Harbor, NY. pp. 59–79.

...tion of Chromosomal Abnormalities
...res ...ence *In Situ* Hybridization Procedures

M. Ke .pski

1. Introduction
1.1. *Fluorescence* In Situ *Hybridization (FISH)*

Cytogenetic changes are important in understanding the pathogenesis of disease. Karyotypic analysis is particularly useful when investigating conditions such as human malignancies, where aneuploidy and structural chromosome rearrangements are commonly found, as in the human leukemias. In these, karyotypes can show a wide range of different structural rearrangements, with highly specific chromosome abnormalities that are used in the classification of leukemias *(1)*, which, in turn, are related to specific clinical features.

Although G-band analysis is traditionally used to detect cytogenetic changes in metaphase chromosomes from tumor tissue, this may occasionally be difficult to interpret where poor chromosome morphology is a feature of disease.

A recent advance in the location and determination of chromosomal abnormalities has been that of fluorescence *in situ* hybridization (FISH), a practical technique for demonstrating the location of specific nucleic acid sequences in individual metaphase and interphase cells *(2,3)*. This procedure is applied alone and in combination with cytogenetic and molecular genetic analysis *(4,5)* for detection and characterization of genetic abnormalities associated with genetic disease *(6,7)* and for the study of radiation biology *(8)* and cancer treatment *(9,10)*. FISH is particularly useful for analysis of cell to cell and intracellular genetic heterogeneity within tumors *(11)*, and it assists detection of rare events such as disseminated metastatic cells (e.g., in the liver and bone marrow). In addition, as FISH has proven to be a sufficiently reliable method, it is being applied in clinical settings, to archived material and to the small amounts of tissue collected during needle biopsy.

From: *Methods in Molecular Medicine, Molecular Diagnosis of Cancer*
Edited by: F. E. Cotter Humana Press Inc., Totowa, NJ

Another novel application of FISH is that of comparative genomic hybridization (CGH), where genomic DNA from tumor cells is hybridized with genomic DNA from normal tissue to normal human metaphase chromosomes to determine changes in sequence copy numbers as gains (amplification) or losses (deletions). This latter procedure is an exciting approach, which is still in its inception, but which has the potential of whole genome analysis in one experiment.

2. Materials

Solutions, glass- and plastic-ware should be sterile.

2.1. Metaphase Preparation

1. 100 mL 1X RPMI-1640 medium (Dutch Modification).
2. 20 mL 1X Fetal calf serum (heat inactivated).
3. 1 mL 200 mM (100X) l-Glutamine.
4. 1 mL 10,000 IU/mL Gentamycin solution.
5. Phytohemagglutinin (PHA).
6. 10 mg/mL Colcemid working solution.
7. 0.075M KCl (5.5 g in 1 L of distilled water).
8. 3:1 Parts absolute methanol:glacial acetic acid fixative, freshly prepared and refrigerated before use.

2.2. Probe Preparation

2.2.1. Nick Translation

1. Probe DNA.
2. dNTP mix (containing 0.2 mM dCTP, 0.2 mM dGTP, 0.2 mM dTTP, 0.1 mM dATP, 0.1 mM Bio-14-dATP or 0.2 mM dCTP, 0.2 mM dGTP, 0.2 mM dATP, 0.1 mM dTTP, 0.1 mM Dig-11-dUTP).
3. Sterile distilled H_2O.
4. Enzyme mix (DNase/Polymerase I) from Gibco, BRL Bionick kit.
5. *E. coli* tRNA.
6. Sonicated herring sperm DNA.
7. 3M Sodium acetate, pH 5.6.
8. Ice-cold ethanol.
9. TE: 10 mM Tris-HCl, pH 8.0, 1 mM EDTA.
10. BRL Bionick kit (Gibco, Paisley, Scotland).

2.2.2. Prehybridization and Hybridization

1. Human Cot-1 DNA.
2. Absolute ice-cold ethanol.
3. Hybridization mix: 50% formamide, 10% dextran sulfate, 1% Tween-20, and 2X SSC.
4. 70% Formamide, 2X SSC (w/v).
5. 70, 85, 100% ice-cold ethanol.
6. Prepared slides, coverslips.

2.2.3. Posthybridization Washes and Signal Detection

1. Formamide solutions (stringency dependent on type of probe): 2X SSC (w/v) 50% formamide, 2X SSC (w/v) 60% formamide.
2. 2X SSC.
3. ST: 4X SSC, 0.05% Tween-20.
4. STB: 4X SSC, 0.05% Tween-20, 3% BSA.
5. Avidin-FITC: 5 mg/mL in STB.
6. Biotinylated anti-avidin: 5 mg/mL in STB.
7. Antidigoxigenin-rhodamine: 5 mg/mL in STB.
8. Citifluor glycerol mountant.
9. Counterstain: 4', 6-Diamidino-2-phenylindole dihydrochloride (DAPI) 2 mg/mL or propidium iodide, 0.5 mg/mL.

2.2.4. Slide Preparation and Pretreatment

1. 1% Decon 90 solution diluted in distilled water.
2. 2X SSC.
3. Proteinase K/$CaCl_2$ solution (10 mg/mL of each in distilled water).

Note: The hybridization buffers, prehybridization, and wash solutions contain formamide, a teratogen. When employing reagents such as formamide and DAPI, caution should be exercised during use. Swallowing, inhalation and absorption through the skin should be avoided. Therefore, good laboratory practice should not include mouth pipeting; and gloves, safety glasses and labcoats should be worn. Universal precautions apply.

3. Methods

During sample preparation for FISH, cells are treated to facilitate disruption of the cell membrane. The nuclei and their chromosomes are then deposited on microscope slides. A probe mixture is subsequently hybridized to the target DNA in the cells affixed to the slides. After hybridization is complete, unbound probe is removed with a series of washes. The methods of sample preparation and fluorescence microscopy will affect hybridization and detection results.

DNA probes used for performing FISH contain a label that allows their detection after hybridization to the target of interest. These probes may be labeled in one of two ways. The direct-labeled probe is the more advanced and simplest to use. A direct-labeled probe is prelabeled with a fluorochrome that allows the fluorescent signal to be bound to the target in one hybridization step (Fig. 1). The alternate method of labeling a probe for FISH application is by using an indirect method, where the DNA probe is prelabeled with a hapten (e.g., Biotin or Digoxigenin). After the hapten-conjugated DNA probe hybridizes to the target sequences, fluorochrome-labeled antibodies to the hapten are used for probe detection (Fig. 2). Alternatively a biotin/streptavidin conjugate is employed (Fig. 3). In either approach, the indirect method relies on a "sand-

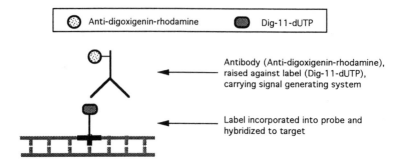

Fig. 1. Signal generating system for immunocytochemical detection of digoxigenin-labeled probe: a one-step detection system.

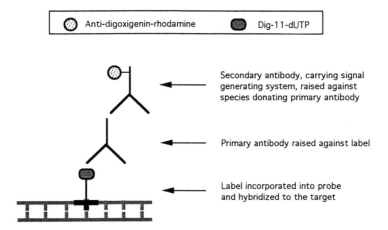

Fig. 2. Signal generating system for immunocytochemical detection using a two-step detection system.

wiching" method, which is more technically awkward because a series of posthybridization steps are required for signal amplification.

The indirect method is a preferred method when hybridizing probes less than 40 kb in size. The direct procedure is the optimal method when labeling DNA for use in comparative genomic hybridization, as it provides a more consistent labeling pattern.

3.1. Metaphase Preparation

The highest quality interphase and metaphase preparations are necessary for effective DNA:DNA *in situ* hybridization (ISH). Residual cytoplasm and other

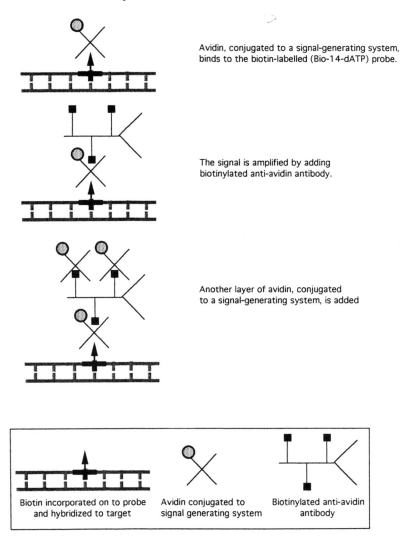

Avidin, conjugated to a signal-generating system, binds to the biotin-labelled (Bio-14-dATP) probe.

The signal is amplified by adding biotinylated anti-avidin antibody.

Another layer of avidin, conjugated to a signal-generating system, is added

| Biotin incorporated on to probe and hybridized to target | Avidin conjugated to signal generating system | Biotinylated anti-avidin antibody |

Fig. 3. Detection of biotin-labeled probes using the biotin-avidin system.

cellular material severely reduce the ISH signal and generate high levels of background signalling. Suitable preparations should show little or no contact between cells, with the density being such that cell location is expedited. However, this may not always be possible, particularly in samples from tumors where cells are known to have notoriously poor morphology, as in the acute lymphoblastic leukemias. Acceptable chromosome spreads should appear with high contrast when examine dry on a microscope slide under phase-contrast.

3.1.1. Metaphase Preparations from Bone Marrow Samples

Bone marrow is a tissue consisting of an unsynchronized population of cells and is treated as direct (1–2 h), overnight (12–24 h), or short-term (48 h) in culture.

1. To 10 mL of complete culture medium, add the following: 100 mL RPMI-1640 medium, 20 mL fetal calf serum (heat inactivated), 1 mL l-Glutamine (20 mM), and 1 mL Gentamycin solution (10,000 IU/mL). Add an appropriate amount of bone marrow to give a final concentration of 10^6 cells/mL.
2. a. Direct cultures: Add 0.1 mL colcemid to give a final concentration of 0.02 mg/mL, and incubate at 37°C for 1 h.
   b. Overnight cultures: Incubate for 12–24 h overnight. One hour prior to harvesting, add 0.1 mL colcemid.
   c. Short-term cultures: Add colcemid as above at 47 h into culture and incubate for an additional hour.
3. Centrifuge the culture at 1300g for 10 min and carefully remove the supernatant.
4. Resuspend the pellet in 10 mL KCl solution by gentle pipeting and leave to stand at room temperature for 15 min.
5. Centrifuge for 6 min at 1300g and remove the supernatant.
6. Add chilled fixative, gradually, up to 5 mL.
7. Repeat steps 5 and 6 twice, reducing the amount of fixative by 2 mL after each spin.
8. Cell suspensions may be stored at –20°C until required.

3.1.2. Metaphase Preparations from Stimulated Peripheral Blood Samples

1. To 10 mL of complete culture medium, add an appropriate amount of peripheral blood to give a final concentration of 10^6 cells/mL.
2. Add 0.2 mL PHA to each culture and incubate at 37°C for 71 h.
3. Add 0.1 mL colcemid and incubate the cultures for an additional 45 min.
4. Samples are then process as in Section 3.1.1.

Excellent detailed protocols on these procedures are provided in Human Cytogenetics II, by B. Czepulkowski et al. *(12)*.

3.1.3. Slide Preparation

The purpose of preparing slides is to produce well-spread chromosomes that remain intact as complete metaphase spreads. Careful slide preparation will also aid in reducing background contamination and therefore nonspecific binding of the probe.

1. Thoroughly clean slides by soaking in a solution of hot water containing 1% Decon 90 for 20 min.
2. Wash slides for 1 h in hot running water, agitating occasionally.
3. Store slides in refrigerated distilled water until ready for use.
4. Release 1–2 drops of cell suspension from a distance of 12–36 in. onto the cold wet slides held at an angle of 30°.

5. Immediately place the slides on a preheated hotplate for a few seconds, allowing evaporation of the water and spreading of the fixed cells. Do not leave the slides on the hotplate for more than a few seconds, as this can result in poor hybridization.
6. Store slides in a sealed container for up to 14 d. Slides may be adequately hybridized after overnight storage.

3.2. Probe Preparation

The diverse types of DNA probes useful in research and for clinical applications can be categorized according to the complexity of the respective target sequences. These range from whole chromosome paints to bacteriophage probes as small as 9 kb in size. Locus specific repeated sequences such as the alphoid cetromeric repeats, or degenerate oligonucleotide primed polymerase chain reaction (DOP-PCR) amplified and labeled whole chromosome paints, are available commercially (Oncor and Cambio). Unique sequences, such as genomic DNA fragments cloned in plasmid (1 kb), phage (9–23 kb), cosmid (40 kb) vectors, or yeast artificial chromosomes (YACs) (200 kb-1 Mb), can be localized against normal or abnormal chromosomes. The minimum size limit for credible detection is approx 3–5 kb, although hybridization using probes under 1 kb in length have been described (13).

3.2.1. Whole Chromosome Paints

Whole chromosome paints (WCPs) are DNA probes that are homologous to DNA sequences along the entire length of the target chromosome (Fig. 4.1). Any one WCP is a mixture of probes for unique DNA sequences on a particular chromosome and are prepared from flow sorted or microdissected, purified human chromosomes. PCR amplified whole chromosome probes have been produced for both human *(14)* and rodent chromosomes *(15)*. Whole chromosome probes are useful for analysis of translocations and particularly for complex cytogenetic rearrangements in metaphase spreads (Figs. 4.2,4.3). Their use on interphase cells is severely limited.

WCPs are prepared and hybridized according to manufacturer's instructions, which are provided with commercially bought probes (Cambio, Oncor). Paints are available both as FITC-and biotin-labeled and therefore can be used in conjunction with each other. Directly-labeled Vysis paints are also now obtainable (Cambio, Oncor).

3.2.2. Centromere Probes

Centromere probes consist of chromosome-specific sequences from highly repetitive human satellite DNA sequences (in most cases, the alpha-satellite sequences located in the centromeric regions). These probes contain no interspersed repeated sequences and the hybridization target is large, often >1 Mb.

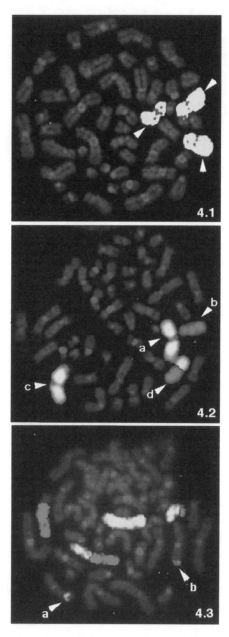

Fig. 4 (*see* color plate number 1 after p. 178). The application of whole chromosome paints for the identification of chromosome rearrangement. **(4.1)** Whole chromosome paint probe. Whole chromosome paint for X (arrowed) showing three copies of chromosome X. **(4.2)** Detection of a chromosome rearrangement using whole chromosome paints. Whole chromosome paints for chromosomes 1 (yellow) and 8 (red) showing: a,

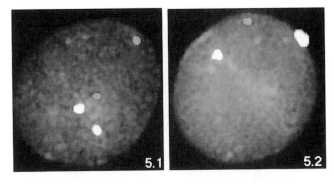

Fig. 5 (*see* color plate number 4 after p. 178). Alpha-satellite centromeric probes used for detection of aneuploidy in interphase cells. **(5.1)** Nonclonal cell showing two signals both for the normal control probe (yellow signal) and for chromosome 7 (red signal). **(5.2)** Clonal cell monosomic for chromosome 7 showing two copies of the control chromosome (yellow signal) and only one copy of chromosome 7 (red signal).

Hybridization is simple, as the signal is large and tightly localized, even in interphase. Chromosome-specific repeat sequence probes are available commercially for all human chromosomes. They are particularly effective for detection of aneusomy in interphase cells (Fig. 5) and for identification of small marker chromosomes *(16)*.

As with WCPs, alpha-satellite probes are available commercially (Cambio, Oncor), both as directly- and indirectly-labeled.

3.2.3. Locus-Specific Probes

Locus-specific probes are usually collections of one or a few cloned sequences homologous to specific human chromosome loci. Hybridization has been performed successfully using probes to targets shorter than 1 kb (cDNA clones) and to larger regions using probes cloned into large insert vectors such as phage (Fig. 6.1), cosmid (Fig. 6.2), and yeast artificial chromosomes (Figs. 6.3[i],[ii]). Hybridization of interspersed repeats in these clones is competi-

---

normal chromosome 1; b, normal chromosome 8; c, derivative chromosome 1 with unknown partner chromosome; and d, derivative chromosome 8, translocated with chromosome 1. **(4.3)** Detection of complex chromosome translocations using whole chromosome paints. Whole chromosome paints for chromosome 4 (yellow) and chromosome 11 (red) showing the involvement of two further chromosomes in: a, by insertion of a portion of chromosome 4 into an unidentified chromosome; and b, a translocated telomeric portion of chromosome 11 onto an unidentified partner chromosome.

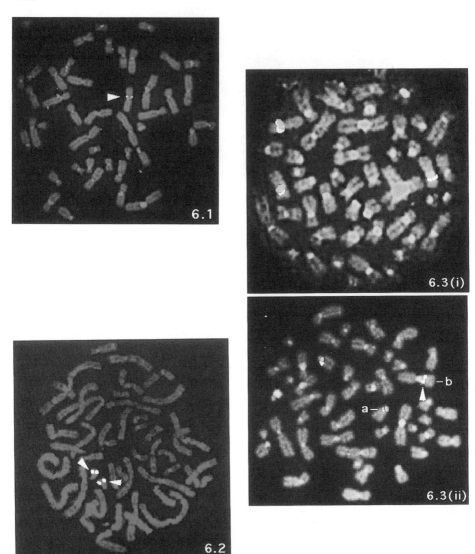

Fig. 6 (*see* color plate number 5 after p. 178). Phage, cosmid, and YAC probes. Yellow signals represent biotin-labeled locus-specific probe. Red signals represent digoxigenin-labeled probe for centromeric region of chromosome X. **(6.1)** Metaphase spread of male cell showing phage probe for region Xp11. Here is an example of a 1.2-kb sized locus-specific probe. This illustrates that detection of minute-sized probes is possible when hybridization conditions are kept at optimal levels. **(6.2)** Cosmid locus-specific probe for the DSCR region of chromosome 21. A Cosmid locus-specific probe for the DSCR region on chromosome 21 at 21q22.3 is clearly seen hybridized to both homologues of chromosome 21 (arrowed). **(6.3)** (i) Metaphase cell showing three copies of chromo-

tively inhibited by applying protocols in which the signals derived from such ubiquitous sequences are suppressed *(17)*. Such a hybridization can be suppressed in a prehybridization reassociation with Cot-1 DNA, which, as a competitor, only uses a reassociation time of 15 min. Such competitive *in situ* suppression means that large segments of the genome can be used as specific probes.

To reach the proficiency needed for diagnostic applications, probes comprising at least 20–50 kb (cosmid-size probes) are required.

3.2.4. Fluorescent Labels

3.2.4.1. BIOTIN

Biotin (vitamin H), found in egg white, is incorporated into the nucleic acid most commonly in the form of biotin-11-dUTP. Biotin-11-dUTP is the most frequently used biotin derivative, but other modified nucleotides are now available, such as biotin-16-dUTP, biotin-14-dATP, and biotin-11-dCTP (Enzo Diagnostics, Sigma, Boehringer Mannheim).

The nucleotides are individually modified at a position that does not interfere with hydrogen bonding between the probe and the target nucleic acid. Also, each contains a linker arm of a minimum of 11 carbon atoms to secure access of the detection reagents and to reduce steric hindrance during probe hybridization.

3.2.4.2. DIGOXIGENIN

Digoxigenin is a steroid that occurs naturally in the plants *Digitalis purpura* and *Digitalis lanata*. Digoxigenin is commonly incorporated into the DNA enzymatically by using the nucleotide derivative digoxigenin-11-dUTP (Boehringer Mannheim).

---

some X: This cell is from a bone marrow sample taken from a child with acute myeloid leukemia, whose normal cells showed two copies of chromosome X, but whose clonal cells carried three copies of chromosome X. G-band analysis suggested the possibility of an inversion within one of the copies of X. However, a YAC probe specific for Xp11 (yellow signal) used in conjunction with an α-satellite probe for X (red signal), showed no inversion within the third chromosome X. (ii) Metaphase cell showing a translocation between chromosomes 1 and 13: A YAC probe specific for the q11 region of chromosome 13 (yellow signal) is seen to have been split, with the remaining portion of the YAC translocated to chromosome 1. (a) The derivative chromosome 13, identified using an α-satellite for 13 (red signal), displaying a smaller signal for the YAC probe, whereas the derivative chromosome 1 also shows a distinct signal for the YAC demonstrating that this probe crosses the breakpoint in the translocation between chromosomes 1 and 13.

3.2.5. Nick Translation

Fluorescent techniques are successfully used in labeling nucleic acids by incorporating DNA using an enzymatic labeling system such as nick translation, which synthesizes labeled nucleic acids using modified nucleotides. This method usually results in the high incorporation of modified nucleotides, thereby generating significantly sensitive probes. Nick translation has been optimized to produce a fragmented probe length suitable for ISH.

The nick translation reaction uses two enzymes, DNase I and *Escherichia coli* DNA polymerase, which incorporate labeled nucleotides along both strands of the DNA duplex (Fig. 7). The most important parameter in the reaction is the action DNase I, which "nicks" double-stranded DNA. Insufficient nicking can lead to inadequate incorporation of the label and probes that are too long. Excessive nicking succeeds only in producing probes that are too short.

1. Using BRL's Bionick kit, add the following to a 1.5-mL microfuge tube on ice: 1 µg probe DNA (phage, cosmid, or YAC), 5 µL dNTP mix (includes Bio-14-dATP),* distilled H_2O to 45 µL, and 5 µL enzyme mix. *For labeling of probes with digoxigenin, exchange the dNTP mix with:

10X digoxigenin-mix	in 100 µL:
0.2 mM dCTP	2 µL of 10 mM
02 mM dGTP	2 µL of 10 mM
0.2 mM dATP	2 µL of 10 mM
0.1 mM dTTP	1 µL of 10 mM
0.1 mM Dig-11-dUTP	10 µL of 1 mM
500 mM Tris-HCl, pH 7.8	50 µL of 1M
50 mM MgCl$_2$	5 µL of 1M
100 mM β-mercaptoethanol	10 µL of 1M
100 mg/mL BSA	10 µL of 1 mg/mL
	8 µL H_2O

2. Incubate at 16°C for 1 h.
3. Add 5 µL stop buffer.
4. The probe may then be purified through a sephadex G50/TE column (this optional, as the probe should be suitably pure if all steps have been followed precisely and the starter probe DNA was pristinely clean).
5. Add 50 µg *E. coli* tRNA and 50 µg herring sperm DNA as carriers to the probe mix.
6. Precipitate the DNA by adding 0.1 vol of 3M NaAc pH 5.6 and 2 vol of ice-cold ethanol.
7. Freeze at −70°C for 15 min or at −20°C for 2 h.
8. Pellet the precipitated DNA at 14,200g for 15 min, dry, and resuspend in 50 µL TE. At this stage, the labeled probe may be stored at −20°C until required.

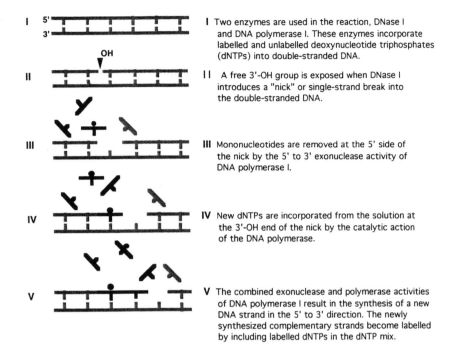

I Two enzymes are used in the reaction, DNase I and DNA polymerase I. These enzymes incorporate labelled and unlabelled deoxynucleotide triphosphates (dNTPs) into double-stranded DNA.

II A free 3'-OH group is exposed when DNase I introduces a "nick" or single-strand break into the double-stranded DNA.

III Mononucleotides are removed at the 5' side of the nick by the 5' to 3' exonuclease activity of DNA polymerase I.

IV New dNTPs are incorporated from the solution at the 3'-OH end of the nick by the catalytic action of the DNA polymerase.

V The combined exonuclease and polymerase activities of DNA polymerase I result in the synthesis of a new DNA strand in the 5' to 3' direction. The newly synthesized complementary strands become labelled by including labelled dNTPs in the dNTP mix.

Fig. 7. The nick translation system.

3.2.6. Prehybridization

The addition of Cot 1 DNA as a blocking or competitor DNA, prior to hybridization, greatly improves signal clarity. The blocking DNA hybridizes to common sequences in the probe and on the chromosomes, thereby preventing hybridization of the probe to these sequences. Only sequences specific to the target are available for probe hybridization *in situ*. The blocking DNA may also prevent hybridization of probe DNA to adjacent DNA sequences by steric hindrance. This method maximizes the rapid reassociation of highly repeated sequences that are common to the probe and to the blocking DNA.

Blocking DNA also hybridizes to molecules in the nucleoplasm and cytoplasm, which could diversely bind probe or detection reagents, leading to undesirable levels of nonspecific binding.

Each hybridization ordinarily occupies an area of the slide 22 × 22 mm (half of a slide). This area should be clearly indicated using a diamond marker. A 100-ng quantity of labeled DNA is necessary for whole slide.

1. Add to each 100 ng of labeled DNA: 2.5 µg Cot 1 DNA and 2 vol ice-cold ethanol.
2. Precipitate for 2 h (or overnight) at −20°C; pellet and dry.

3. Resuspend the pellet in an appropriate quantity of hybridization mix (need 20–30 μL/slide). (The probe may again be stored at –20°C at this stage until required.)
4. Denature probe mix at 70°C for 5 min and cool by plunging briefly into ice.
5. Pulse spin to ensure all liquid is at the base of the tube; preanneal at 37°C for 1–3 h. (While the probe is preannealing, continue with slide pretreatment and preparation in Section 3.3.)

3.3. Pretreatment and Slide Preparation

Before ISH, material is pretreated to reduce nonspecific probe hybridization to nontarget nucleic acids and to reduce nonspecific association with proteins or other elements that may bind the probe. This procedure also aids probe and detection reagent penetration and maintains the stability of target sequences.

Chromosomal DNA from the cells on the slide are denatured (rendered single-stranded) to allow hybridization with the fluorescently labeled probe.

3.3.1. Pretreatment of Slides

Incubate slides in 2X SSC at 37°C for 30–60 min.

3.3.2. Denaturation and Preparation of Slides for Hybridization

1. Immerse slides into Coplin jars containing 70% formamide, 2X SSC at 70°C for 2 min.
2. After 2 min incubation, remove the slides using forceps and proceed immediately to the ice-cold ethanol washes. Agitate the slides slightly at the start of each wash: 70% ethanol for 2 min, 85% ethanol for 2 min, and 100% ethanol for 2 min.
3. Air-dry slides for 5 min.
4. Place dried slides into a Proteinase K/CaCl$_2$ solution at room temperature for 8 min.
5. Transfer to the ice-cold ethanol series as in step 2.
6. Air dry for 5 min.

3.4. Hybridization

1. Place slides on a warm hotplate (37°C); meanwhile spin preannealed probe briefly.
2. Apply probe to prewarmed slide and add a coverslip, avoiding air bubbles.
3. Seal hybridization area with rubber cement and incubate at 37°C for 24–48 h in a moist chamber.

3.5. Detection and Posthybridization Washes

Posthybridization washes are normally carried out in a slightly more stringent solution than the hybridization mixture to denature and remove weakly bound probe, leaving predominantly positively matched nucleotides in the duplex. It is important that slides are not allowed to dry at any stage.

Most probe labels are immunogenic and are detected by antibodies raised against the label. Digoxigenin uses a system that involves conjugation to the primary antibody (raised against the label) in a one-step detection method (Fig. 1). Biotin has two detection systems, either antibiotin or the biotin-(strept)avidin system.

Avidin is glycoprotein extracted from egg white, which has a significant affinity for biotin. The first step in the detection of biotin is the addition of avidin conjugated to a signal-generating system (Fig. 3). The signal is then amplified by using biotinylated anti-avidin (an antibody raised against avidin, conjugated to biotin) followed by a further layer of avidin conjugated to the signal-generating system.

3.5.1. Posthybridization Washes

1. Prepare the detection reagents as follows:
   a. For the detection of digoxigenin-labeled signals: 2.5 µL of antidigoxigenin-rhodamine in 1 mL STB.
   b. For the detection of biotin-labeled signals: 2.5 mL of avidin in 1 mL STB and 10 µL of biotinylated anti-avidin in 1 mL STB.
2. Remove coverslip by flicking off the slide carefully. Ensure that the coverslip is not removed by sliding off the slide as this may cause distortion of material and signal. Do not allow slides to dry at any stage prior to counterstaining and mounting.
3. Wash slides as follows at 43°C: 3X in 50% formamide, 2X SSC (w/v) (5 min); 3X in 2X SSC (5 min). All remaining washes are carried out at room temperature.
4. Proceed to wash slides as follows: 1X in 4X SSC, 0.05% Tween-20 (ST) (3 min); 1X in 4X SSC, 0.05% Tween-20, 3% BSA (STB) (10 min); 1X in 4X SSC, 0.05% Tween-20 (ST) (3 min).

3.5.2. Signal Detection

1. Incubate slides, in the dark,* by depositing 100 µL of avidin per slide and applying a coverslip to prevent drying of the slide during incubation. Leave for 20 min. (*Fluorescein is readily photobleached).
2. Slide off the coverslips and wash as follows: 3X in ST (3 min).
3. Incubate slides as in step 1, detecting with biotinylated anti-avidin. Leave to incubate for 20 min.
4. Wash as in step 2.
5. Repeat steps 1 and 2 once more.
6. At this stage, the slides can be mounted or dehydrated in ethanol and stored.

3.5.3. Counterstaining of Slides

1. Slides should be mounted in "Citifluor," containing a counterstain (either Propidium iodide [0.5 mg/mL] or DAPI [2 mg/mL]) by depositing one drop on each slide and applying a 25 × 50 mm coverslip.
2. Allow slides to stand for 5 min.
3. Carefully blot each slide firmly, to secure the coverslip and seal with rubber cement. Mounted slides may be kept at 4°C for at least 6 mo.

3.5.4. Analysis for FISH

For light microscopic analysis, the method chosen is limited to the type of signal-generating system used for detecting the in situ signal. The aim of any system is the localization of the hybridization signal with the maximum sensitivity and spatial resolution possible.

Analysis of chromosome translocations, using whole chromosome paints, can be successfully effected using a simple epifluorescence microscope with the appropriate filters. However, for detection of smaller signals, from phage and cosmid probes, or indeed YACs crossing translocation breakpoints, rather more sophisticated equipment is necessary for detailed FISH analysis.

The confocal scanning optical microscope allows noninvasive optical sectioning, thereby removing the presence of distorted (out of focus) images generated by conventional epifluorescence microscopy, which interferes with the image. Confocal microscopy is now used routinely by many laboratories for imaging two-dimensional material such as metaphase spreads and interphase nuclei, which sustain ISH signals. However, the only disadvantage in using this type of system exists in the lack of an image-processing facility.

Digital imaging systems are now widely available that allow the recording of images electronically by using video or low-light cameras. These are highly sophisticated devices using a combination of microscope, camera, and computer with advanced software. There has been a growing demand to make this technology available to scientists without specialized image processing knowledge. Several companies have addressed this problem with the subsequent creation of appropriate software designed to capture, analyze, and process FISH images. The illustrations included in this chapter have all been processed using a Photometrics camera and SmartCapture software (Digital Scientific). This software is compatible with all models of Macintosh.

The SmartCapture imaging system allows visualization of fluorescent signals from a fluorescent microscope. The systems has the capacity to image and determine faint FISH signals with remarkable clarity. This arrangement combines a high-performance, digital charged-couple device (CCD) camera with powerful imaging software to allow appropriation and analysis of even the weakest signals. Resolution of the Photometrics CCD camera approximates the theoretical maximum for light, making SmartCapture one of the most powerfully sensitive FISH imaging systems available. The system creates a 24-bit color image with maximum signal intensity.

The material under investigation is located and focused by eye and the image is then amassed and recorded over several seconds by the CCD camera and presented on the computer monitor. If signals are very weak, the time required to search and record images in each field of view may be taxing; however, the results are undeniably worthwhile. The advantage of the CCD system is that ISH signals do not have to be greatly amplified to enable visualization. This inevitably induces higher sensitivity and resolution.

4. Notes

1. Applications of FISH procedures. The rapidity and flexibility of FISH methods lend themselves for use, not only in research, but in assisting clinical diagnosis. This is particularly valuable in assessing minimal residual disease after chemo- or radiotherapy and also in the speedy cytogenetic evaluation of a relapse sample for the presence or absence of a known clonal abnormality. Both centromeric probes and WCPs are conducive for confirming cytogenetic status in such clinical inquires.

2. Acute leukemias. In acute myeloid leukemias, specific numerical abnormalities, namely a loss of chromosome 7 (Fig. 5) or a gain of chromosome 8, are amongst the most common cytogenetic changes in AML *(18,19)*. These are easily detected by FISH using chromosome-specific repeat sequence probes. High hybridization efficiencies can be achieved on clinical material such a blood or bone marrow smears *(20,21)*. The application of FISH for the detection of the most common translocation in AML, the t(8;21) *(22)*, t(15;17) *(23)*, inv(16) *(24)*, and 11q23 abnormalities *(25)*, has been shown; however, to date, no study has been published evaluating these for routine clinical use.

   Although numerical changes occur in acute lymphoblastic leukemia in similar frequencies as in AML, no systematic study confronting these abnormalities in ALL has been published to date. The most common chromosomal translocation in adult ALL is the t(9;22)(q34;q11). a probe set is commercially available (Oncor) for the detection of the bcr-abl fusion (Fig. 8), the molecular complement of the t(9;22), in ALL. It is based on a yeast artificial chromosome probe spanning both the major and the minor breakpoint cluster regions of the BCR gene.

3. Loss of heterozygosity. Wilms' tumor is an embryonal malignancy of the kidney that affects about 1 in 10,000 infants and young children. It can occur in both sporadic and familial forms. A subset of Wilms' tumor cases occurs in association with aniridia, genito-urinary abnormalities, and mental retardation, known as the WAGR syndrome. Although familial cases of WAGR syndrome are rare, patients frequently have a cytogenetically detectable deletion on the short arm of chromosome 11 that has been mapped to 11p13.

   Similarly in retinoblastoma (an intraocular cancer predominantly found in young children, with an incidence of approx 1 in 20,000), a detectable deletion on the long arm of chromosome 13 at 13q14 has frequently been observed. Cosmid probes for Rb and WT1 are available and are useful for the rapid detection of loss of heterozygosity in either of these conditions (Figs. 9 and 10).

4. Monitoring treatment outcome. Dual-color hybridization with X and Y chromosome-specific centromeric probes is a successful approach to sexing interphase cells following bone-marrow transplantation between sex-mismatched patient and donor. This procedure enables the effective monitoring of engraftment of donor cells (Fig. 11).

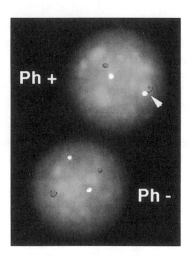

Fig. 8 (*see* color plate number 2 after p. 178). Interphase cells from a patient with chronic myelogenous leukemia. Cosmid probes for the **abl** locus on chromosome 9 (yellow signal) and for the **bcr** locus on chromosome 22 (red signal) show the presence of a Philadelphia translocation (arrowed) in the Philadelphia +ive cell. The Philadelphia −ive cell shows two distinct signals for the **abl** locus and two distinct signals for the **bcr** locus.

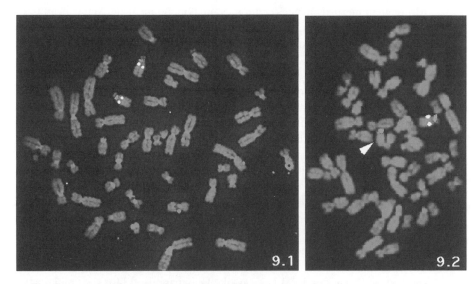

Fig. 9 (*see* color plate number 6 after p. 178). The detection of loss of heterozygosity in retinoblastoma. **(9.1)** Normal control cell hybridized with a cosmid probe (yellow signal) for the Rb region on chromosome 13 at 13q14. Both copies of chromosome 13 carry signals for the Rb gene locus. An α-satellite probe for 13 (green signal) is used to identify both homologs. **(9.2)** Metaphase cell from a patient with retinoblastoma showing loss of heterozygosity for the Rb region of chromosome 13 (arrowed). The homolog with the Rb deletion is identified using a cetromeric probe specific for chromosome 13 (green signal).

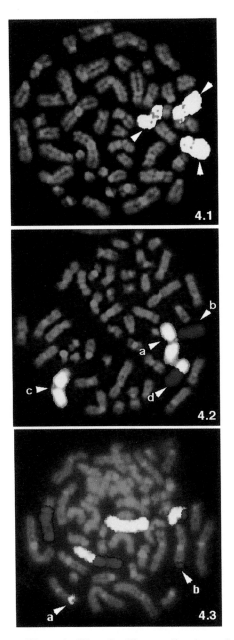

4.1

4.2

4.3

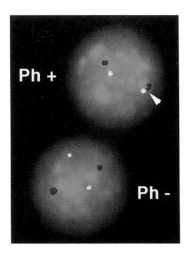

Ph +

Ph -

Plate 2 (Fig. 8). Interphase cells from a patient with chronic myelogenous leukemia. *See* full caption on p. 178 and discussion in Chapter 13.

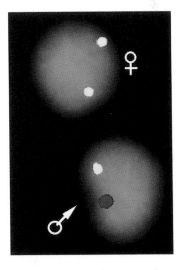

♀

♂

Plate 1 (Fig. 4). The application of whole chromosome paints for the identification of chromosome rearrangement. *See* full caption on p. 168 and discussion in Chapter 13.

Plate 3 (Fig. 11). Centromeric probes used following a sex-mismatched bone marrow transplant. *See* full caption on p. 179 and discussion in Chapter 13.

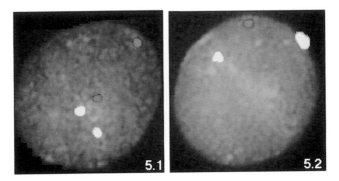

Plate 4 (Fig. 5). Alpha-satellite centromeric probes used for detection of aneuploidy in interphase cells. *See* full caption on p. 169 and discussion in Chapter 13.

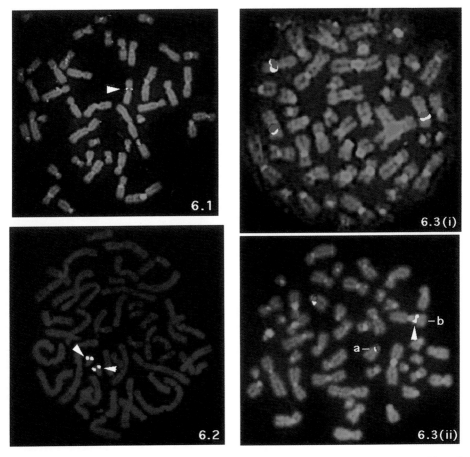

Plate 5 (Fig. 6). Phage, cosmid, and YAC probes. *See* full caption on p. 170 and discussion in Chapter 13.

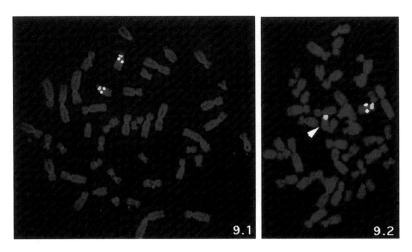

Plate 6 (Fig. 9). The detection of loss of heterozygosity in retinoblastoma. *See* full caption on p. 178 and discussion in Chapter 13.

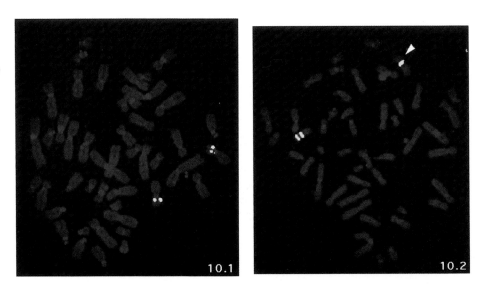

Plate 7 (Fig. 10). The detection of loss of heterozygosity in Wilms' tumor. *See* full caption on p. 179 and discussion in Chapter 13.

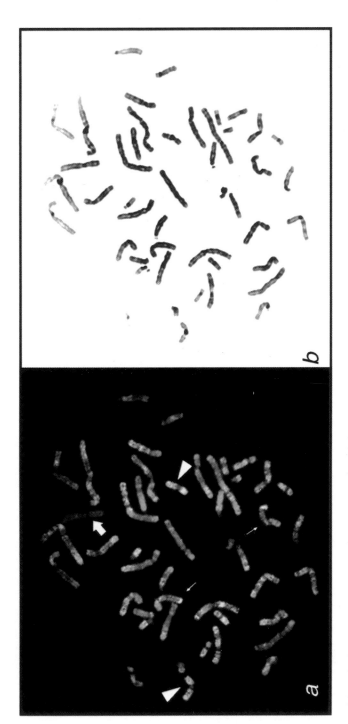

Plate 8 (Fig. 1). (a) Comparative genomic hybridization of a prostate cancer xenograft, LuCAP. **(b)** An inverse DAPI (pseudo-Geisma banding) image of the same metaphase for chromosome identification. *See* full caption on p. 185 and discussion in Chapter 14.

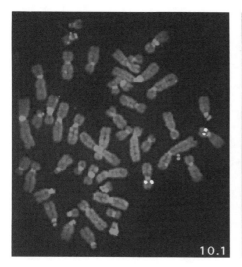
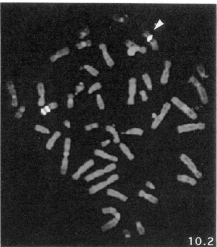

Fig. 10 (*see* color plate number 7 after p. 178). The detection of loss of heterozygosity in Wilms' tumor. **(10.1)** Normal control cell hybridized with a cosmid probe specific for the WT1 region of chromosome 11 at 11p13 (yellow signal). Both homologs for chromosome 11 carry signals for the WT1 locus. **(10.2)** Metaphase cell from a patient with Wilms' tumor showing loss of heterozygosity for the WT1 region in one chromosome 11 (arrowed). The homolog deleted for WT1 is identified with an α-satellite probe specific for chromosome 11 (centromeric yellow signal).

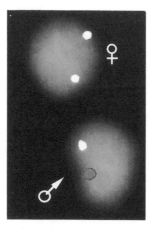

Fig. 11 (*see* color plate number 3 after p. 178). Centromeric probes used following a sex-mismatched bone marrow transplant. Alpha-satellite probes specific for chromosome X (yellow signal) and chromosome Y (red signal) are useful when monitoring engraftment following a transplant where the donor is of the opposite sex to the host. ♀ represents engrafted female donor cell showing two α-satellite signals for chromosome X. ○→ represents male host cell showing one each of α-satellite signals for chromosomes X and Y.

Acknowledgments

Thanks are due to Jane Chalker, Department of Haematology, Great Ormond St. Hospital for Sick Children, London, for providing Fig. 11.

References

1. Sixth International Workshop on Chromosomes in Leukaemia (1989) Six-year follow-up of the clinical significance of karyotype in acute lymphoblastic leukaemia. *Cancer Genet. Cytogenet.* **40,** 171–185.
2. Pinkel, D. and Trask, B. (1990) Fluorescence *in situ* hybridization with DNA probes. *Methods Cell. Biol.* **33,** 383–400.
3. Pinkel, D., Landegent, J., Collins, C., Fuscoe, J., Segraves, R., Lucas, J., and Gray, J. (1988) Fluorescence in situ hybridization with human chromosome-specific libraries: Detection of trisomy 21 and translocations of chromosome 4. *Proc. Natl. Acad. Sci. USA* **85,** 9138–9142.
4. Pinkel, D., Straume, T., and Gray, J. W. (1986) Cytogenetic analysis using quantitative, high-sensitivity fluorescence hybridization. *Proc. Natl. Acad. Sci. USA* **83,** 2934–2938.
5. Le Beau, M., Espinosa, R., Neuman, W. L., Stock, W., Roulston, D., Larson, R. A., Keinanen, M., and Westbrook, C. A. (1993) Cytogenetic and molecular delineation of the smallest commonly deleted region of chromosome 5 in malignant myeloid diseases. *Proc. Natl. Acad. Sci. USA* **90,** 5484–5488.
6. Bentz, M., Schroder, M., Herz, M., Stilgenbauer, S., Lichter, P., and Dohner, H. (1993) Detection of trisomy 8 on blood smears using fluorescence *in situ* hybridization. *Leukemia* **7,** 752–757.
7. Zhang, J., Meltzer, P., Jenkins, R., Guan, X. Y., and Trent, J. (1993) Application of chromosome microdissection probes for elucidation of BCR-ABL fusion and variant Philadelphia chromosome translocations in chronic myelogenous leukemia. *Blood* **81,** 3365–3371.
8. Schmid, E., Zitzelsberger, H., Braselmann, H., Gray, J. and Bauchinger, M. (1992) Radiation-induced chromosome aberrations analysed by fluorescence *in situ* hybridization with a triple combination of composite whole chromosome-specific DNA probes. *Int. J. Rad. Biol.* **62,** 673–678.
9. Anastasi, J., Thangavelu, M., Vardiman, J. W., Hooberman, A. L., Bian, M. L., Larson, R. A., and Le, B. M. (1991) Interphase cytogenetic analysis detects minimal residual disease in a case of acute allogeneic bone marrow transplantation. *Blood* **77,** 1087–1091.
10. Zhao, L., Kantarjian, H. M., Van, O. J., Cork, A., Trujillo, J. M., and Liang, J. C. (1993) Detection of residual proliferating leukemic cells by fluorescence *in situ* hybridization in CML patients in complete remission after interferon treatment. *Leukemia* **7,** 168–171.
11. Sauter, G., Moch, H., Moore, D., Carroll, P., Kerschmann, R., Chew, K., Mihatsch, M. J., Gudat, F., and Waldman, F. (1993) Heterogeneity of erbB-2 gene amplification in bladder cancer. *Cancer Res.* **53,** 2199–2203.

12. Czepulkowski, B. H., Bhatt, B., and Rooney, D. E. (1992) Basic techniques for the preparation and analysis of chromosomes from bone marrow and leukaemic blood, in *Human Cytogenetics II: A Practical Approach* (Rooney, D. E. and Czepulkowski, B. H., eds.), pp. 1–12.
13. Viegas-Pequignot, E., Berrard, S., Brice, A., Apiou, F., and Mallet, J. (1991) Localization of a 900-bp-long fragment of the human choline acetyltransferase gene to 10q11.2 by nonradioactive *in situ* hybridization. *Genomics* **9(1),** 210.
14. Vooijs, M., Yu, L. C., Tkachuk, D., Pinkel, D., Johnson, D., and Gray, J. W. (1993) Libraries for each human chromosome, constructed from sorter-enriched chromosomes by using linker-adaptor PCR. *Am. J. Hum. Genet.* **52,** 586–597.
15. Weier, H.-U., Ploikoff, D., Fawcett, J., Lee, K.-H., Cram, L. S., Chapman, V., and Gray, J. W. (1994) Generation of five high complexity painting probe libraries from flow sorted mouse chromosomes. *Genomics* **21(3),** 641–644.
16. Kiechle, S. M., Decker, H. J., Berger, C. S. Fiebig, H. H., and Sandberg, A. A. (1991) Detection of monosomy in interphase nuclei and identification of marker chromosomes using biotinylated alpha-satellite DNA probes. *Cancer Genet. Cytogenet.* **51,** 23–33.
17. Lichter, P., Cremer, T., Borden, J., Manuelidis, L., and Ward, D. C. (1988) Delineation of individual human chromosomes in metaphase and interphase cells by *in situ* suppression hybridization using recombinant DNA libraries. *Hum. Genet.* 30, 224–234.
18. Berger, R., Bernheim, A., Ochoa-Noguera, M. E., Daniel, M. T., Valensi, F., Sigaux, F., Flandrin, G., and Boiron, M. (1987) Prognostic significance of chromosomal abnormalities in acute nonlymphocytic leukemia: a study of 343 patients. *Cancer Genet. Cytogenet.* **28,** 293–299.
19. Fenaux, P., Preudhomme, C., Lai, J. L., Morel, P., Beuscart, R., and Bautlers, F. (1989) Cytogenetics and their prognostic value in *de novo* acute myeloid leukemia: a report on 283 cases. *Br. J. Haematol.* **73,** 61–67.
20. Bentz, M., Schröder, M., Herz, M., Stilgenbauer, S., Lichter, P., and Dahner, H. (1993) Detection of trisomy 8 on blood smears using fluorescence *in situ* hybridization. *Leukemia* **7,** 752–757.
21. van Lorn, K., Hagemeijer, A., Smit, E. M. E., and Lowenberg, B. (1993) *In situ* hybridization on May-Grünwald-Giemsa-stained bone marrow and blood smears of patients with hematologic disorders allows detection of cell-lineage-specific cytogenetic abnormalities. *Blood* **82,** 884–888.
22. Gao, J. Erickson, P., Gardiner, K., Le Beau, M. M., Diaz, M. O., Patterson, D., Rowley, J. D., and Drabkin, H. A. (1991) Isolation of a yeast artificial chromosome spanning the 8;21 translocation breakpoint t(8;21)(q22;q22.3) in acute myelogenous leukemia. *Proc. Natl. Acad. Sci USA* **88,** 4882–4886.
23. Warrell, R. P., de Thé, H., Wang, Z. Y., and Degos, L. (1993) Acute promyelocytic leukemia. *N. Eng. J. Med.* **329,** 177–189.
24. Dauwerse, J. G. Kievits, T., Beverstock, G. C., van der Keur, D., Smit, E., Wessels, H. W., Hagemeijer, A., Pearson, P. L., van Ommen, G. J. B., and Breuning, M. H. (1990) Rapid detection of chromosome 16 inversion in acute nonlymphocytic leukemia, subtype M4: regional localization of the breakpoint in 16p. *Cytogenet. Cell Genet.* **53,** 126–138.

25. Rowley, J. D., Diaz, M. O., Espinosa, R., III, Patel, Y. D., van Melle, E., Ziemin, S., Taillon-Miller, P., Lichter, P., Evans, G. A., Kersey, J. H., Ward, D. C., Domer, P. H., Le Beau, M. M. (1990) Mapping chromosome band 11q23 in human acute leukemia with biotinylated probes: identification of 11q23 translocation break-points with a yeast artificial chromosome. *Proc. Natl. Acad. Sci. USA* **87,** 9358–9362.
26. Knudson, A. G., Jr. (1985) Hereditary cancer, oncogenes, and antioncogenes. *Cancer Res.* **45,** 1437–1443.

14

Comparative Genomic Hybridization

Briana J. Williams

1. Introduction

Numerical genetic changes can be most easily examined by simply preparing metaphase chromosomes and counting the number of chromosomes in the spread. Unfortunately, it is often impossible to obtain high-quality metaphase preparations from samples, especially solid tumors. Even more frustrating, it is just such tissues that are particularly interesting to study. For example, numerical imbalances in these tumors might identify the sites of either tumor suppressor genes in deleted regions or proto-oncogenes in amplified regions involved in the initiation or progression of that particular disease. A submicroscopic molecular method, such as loss of heterozygosity (LOH) or allelic imbalance (AI), will provide much greater detail in a small region, but is impractical to have that level of detail in a genome-wide screen. Because of these limitations, a novel methodology was needed to evaluate the numerical genetic composition of interesting samples, especially solid tumors.

Comparative genomic hybridization (CGH) was introduced in 1992 for the detection of deletions and amplifications in solid tumors, and the technique is still without rival as a one-step genome-wide screening for such numerical abnormalities *(1)*. In fact, CGH has now been reported for genetic imbalance detection in many different types of solid tumors, leukemias, as well as lymphomas, and for clinical applications such as monosomy/trisomy detection *(2–8)*. In general, CGH is a rather sophisticated application of several very basic fluorescence *in situ* hybridization FISH techniques. In its simplest form, CGH is carried out by labeling a test DNA (i.e., tumor DNA) in one color fluorochrome (i.e., red) and a reference DNA (i.e., normal DNA from lymphocytes) in a second color fluorochrome (i.e., green). CGH is carried out under suppression conditions, and so the oppositely labeled DNAs are mixed with a

From: *Methods in Molecular Medicine, Molecular Diagnosis of Cancer*
Edited by: F. E. Cotter Humana Press Inc., Totowa, NJ

blocking DNA such as Cot-1, denatured, and allowed to preanneal to make the repetitive DNA particularly at the centromeres unavailable for hybridization. The denatured and preannealed DNA mixture is then applied to a slide with normal metaphases, which act as a template for the hybridization. The length of hybridization can be 48–96 h or more. After a rigorous postwashing protocol, the chromosomes are counterstained with DAPI and coverslipped for observation. In chromosomal regions that are present in the same relative copy number in the test and reference DNAs, the resultant FISH signals will be an equal mixture of red and green. In those regions that are not in relative numerical balance (because of abnormalities in the test DNA such as amplifications, deletions or copy number changes of particular chromosomes), the FISH signals will appear either more red (amplifications or increased copy number) or more green (deletions or decreased copy number) than the surrounding regions. A dedicated computer software program and highly sensitive cooled-CCD camera are absolutely necessary to accurately determine the relative fluorescence intensity at each point along the medial axis of every chromosome (*see* Fig. 1). It is possible, however, to visually identify (but not mathematically analyze) large regions of color imbalance or even relatively small amplified regions. Whereas, while CGH is based on some very basic FISH methodologies, its correct technical application and analysis make it less accessible to all laboratories. CGH has some technical limitations that not only require a level of sophistication in sample preparation and analysis, but may make CGH inappropriate for some other clinical applications. For example, CGH cannot detect polyploidy, balanced translocations, inversions, or point mutations. Additionally, CGH is carried out under extreme suppression conditions, making analysis of sequences very near the centromere, telomeres, or heterochromatic regions impossible. The technique has been reported to have successfully detected approximately fourfold to sevenfold genetic amplifications. The deletion detection limit of CGH is approx 10–20 Mb in cell lines and 20–30 Mb in primary tumors (approximately the size of an average chromosomal band). While this provides CGH with essentially the sensitivity of traditional cytogenetic evaluation, it is not limited by the low mitotic index of many tumors. Although, being a DNA-based assay, CGH is seriously limited by a high degree of sample contamination by normal, nontarget cells. The use of paraffin-embedded tissues (PET) for CGH analysis may overcome some of the limitations of cellular heterogeneity as a sample can be carefully microdissected after histological and pathological evaluation. Alternatively, where appropriate, cells may be sorted by flow cytometry.

If very few cells are available, or if using CGH for a single-cell application, PCR-based amplification of the DNA using universal primers may be used *(9,10)*. These methodologies may yield adequate amounts of DNA for CGH,

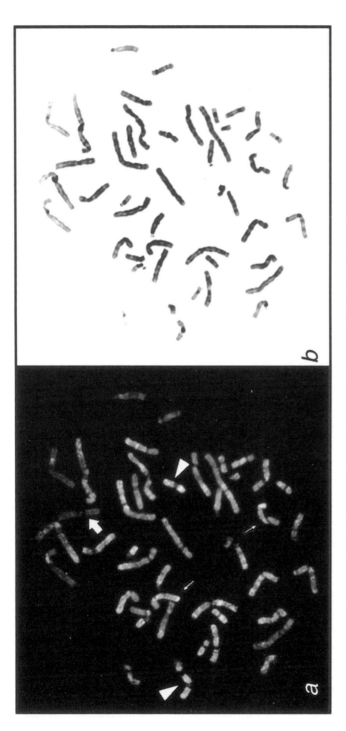

Fig. 1 (*see* color plate number 8 after p. 178). **(A)** Comparative genomic hybridization of a prostate cancer xenograft, LuCAP, kindly provided by Drs. William Ellis and Robert Vessells, University of Washington. The tumor DNA was labeled in Texas Red and the normal reference DNA in FITC (green). The following numerical imbalances were detected after digital analysis using CGH-specific software provided by Vysis Inc., Downers Grove, IL: loss of regions of 2q, 6p, 8p, 9, 10p, 17p, and 18q, and gains of 3p, 3q, 5q, 6q, 7, 8q, 11q, 16q, and the X chromosome. Examples of whole chromosome loss are shown at the arrowheads (chromosomes 9), whole chromosome gain at the large arrow (X chromosome), and loss of p arm and gain of q arm material at the small arrows (chromosomes 8); **(B)** an inverse DAPI (pseudo-Geimsa banding) image of the same metaphase for chromosome identification.

but there is evidence that the amplification may not cover the entire genome or be entirely random, and it may be allele specific at many loci. The minimal technical requirements for both sample preparation and analysis are examined in a number of recent publications *(11–16)*. These should be reviewed before beginning CGH experiments.

2. Materials
2.1. Labeling of DNA by Nick Translation for CGH
1. Texas Red-dUTP (NEN DuPont, Boston, MA).
2. Fluorescein-dUTP (NEN DuPont).
3. Commercially available nick translation kit (Gibco/BRL, Gaithersburg, MD).
4. DNA Polymerase I enzyme (such as from Gibco/BRL).
5. Distilled water.

2.2. Column Chromatography
Sephadex G–50 column, or prepare as follows: 1 cc syringe glass wool, 15-mL conical tube, and TE^{-4} (10 mM Tris-HCl, pH 8.0, 0.1 mM EDTA, pH 8.0).

2.3. Preparation of the DNA Mixture
1. Cot-1 DNA (Gibco/BRL).
2. 1.5-mL microfuge tube.
3. 3M Sodium acetate, pH 5.5.
4. Absolute ethanol.
5. 50% hybridization mixture (such as Hybrisol VII, Oncor, Gaithersburg, MD).
6. Formamide.
7. 2X SSC (pH 7.0).
8. Cold ethanol series (70, 90, and 100%).
9. 22 × 50 mm glass coverslip.
10. Humid chamber.

2.4. Posthybridization Washes
1. 50% Formamide/2X SSC (pH 7.0) at 45°C, 3 jars.
2. 2X SSC (pH 7.0) at 45°C.
3. 2X SSC (pH 7.0) at room temperature.
4. PN buffer: 0.1M NaH$_2$PO$_4$, 0.1M Na$_2$HPO$_4$, 0.05% Nonidet P40, pH 8.2.
5. Distilled water.
6. 2 mg/mL of 4'-Diamidino-2-phenylindole dihydrochloride (DAPI) in antifade solution.
7. 22 × 50 mm glass coverslip.

3. Methods
3.1. Extraction of DNA for CGH
DNA should be high-quality, high-mol-wt DNA extracted using standard extraction techniques or from any number of commercially-available kits. Approximately 200–400 ng of DNA are required for each CGH slide, but a

considerable DNA is lost in the various manipulations. The numerical alterations found in CGH experiments should be verified by repeating the hybridization with the DNAs labeled in the opposite colored fluorochromes (i.e., for experiment 1 red test/green reference and for experiment 2 green test/red reference). Therefore, at least 1.5 µg of DNA should be available for analysis. If using PET samples, additional (up to 4 d, adding enzyme each day) Proteinase K digestion may be required to provide high enough yields.

3.2. Labeling of DNA by Nick Translation for CGH

Label the test and reference DNA with different fluorescent nucleotides, such as Texas Red-dUTP and fluorescein-dUTP (NEN DuPont) using a commercially-available nick translation kit and additional DNA Polymerase I enzyme (such as from Gibco/BRL) to increase the length of the resultant fragments. (The average fragment length should be 1.5–3.0 kb, adjust enzymes as necessary.)

On ice, mix: a volume of DNA to equal 1.5 µg, a volume of dH$_2$O required to make a final volume of 50 µL, 5.0 µL Solution A4 (contains dATP, dCTP, and dGTP), 1.0 µL fluorescent dUTP (either red OR green), 5.0 µL Solution C (enzyme mix containing Polymerase I and DNAse I), and 1.0 µL Polymerase I (holoenzyme). Final 50-µL vol.

1. Quick-spin the tubes and incubate for 1 h at 16°C.
2. After 1 h, add 5 µL stop buffer.
3. Remove unincorporated nucleotides from sample by column chromatography.

3.3. Column Chromatography

The unincorporated nucleotides will create excess background signals and must be removed. Ethanol precipitation is not sufficient for complete removal of the excess label and should not be used. Apply sample to premade Sephadex G-50 column, or prepare as follows:

1. Prepare column by plugging a 1-mL syringe without needle with a small piece of glass wool.
2. Place the syringe in a 15-mL conical tube.
3. Allow a full column of TE^{-4} to run through the plugged syringe.
4. Carefully fill the syringe, from the bottom up, with Sephadex G-50 fine beads pre-swollen with TE^{-4}.
5. After the excess TE has dripped out, spin the column at 90g for 3 min.
6. Remove the excess TE from the tube and carefully load the 55-µL labeled DNA sample to the column (a maximum of 3 tubes can be run over a single column).
7. After the sample has run into the column bed, add an equal volume of TE.
8. Spin exactly as above, and remove eluent to storage tube.
9. The approximate concentration is 14 ng/µL, or it can be more precisely quantitated.

3.4. Preparation of the DNA Mixture

1. Place 200–400 ng of labeled test DNA, an equal concentration of reference DNA and 50 μg of Cot-1 DNA (Gibco/BRL) in a 1.5-mL microfuge tube.
2. Add 0.1 vol of 3*M* sodium acetate, pH 5.5, mix, and add 2.25 vol of absolute ethanol; mix.
3. Centrifuge at >12,500*g* for 30 min.
4. Decant and dry for 15 min.
5. Dissolve pellet in 20 μL 50% hybridization mixture (Hybrisol VII, Oncor).
6. Denature 5–10 min at 73°C, and preanneal at 37°C for 15–60 min.
7. Simultaneously denature slides in 70% formamide, 2X SSC, pH 7.0, for 2 min at 73°C.
8. Dehydrate slides through a cold ethanol series (70, 90, and 100%). Air dry and warm to 37°C.
9. Apply the probe/hybridization mixture to separately denatured slides and coverslip with a 22 × 22 mm glass coverslip. Seal the coverslip in place with rubber cement.
10. Incubate 48–96 h at 37°C in a humid chamber.

3.5. Posthybridization Washes

Each wash takes 10 min at the specified temperature.

1. Washes 1–3: 50% formamide/2X SSC (pH 7.0) at 45°C.
2. Wash 4: 2X SSC, pH 7.0 at 45°C.
3. Wash 5: 2X SSC, pH 7.0 at room temperature.
4. Wash 6: PN buffer at room temperature.
5. Wash 7: Distilled water at room temperature.

Air dry the slide; apply 25 μL DAPI in antifade solution and coverslip with a 22 × 50 mm glass coverslip. Visualize the slide.

3.6. Image Analysis

While some of the numerical changes (particularly amplifications) can be directly visualized, quantitative analysis of CGH results requires a sophisticated software program dedicated specifically to CGH analysis. The specific procedures to follow are unique to each manufacturer's program, but the general concepts are common to all of the systems. The basis for CGH analysis is the separate quantitation of the red signal intensity and green signal intensity and the plotting of these relative to one another at each pixel along the medial axis of each chromosome. In order to accomplish this, the chromosomes must be identified by their DAPI banding pattern, which is technically challenging to those without cytogenetic experience or much practice. Most of the analysis packages available will produce an enhanced "pseudo-Geimsa" banding pattern based on the DAPI staining, which is more helpful for identification. Once the chromosomes are identified, the medial axes may be drawn and the software then calculates the intensity profiles for each chromosome. The information is gathered and pooled over several metaphases and average profiles with standard error measures can be made for each chromosome. Deviations above or below established thresholds signify increases or decreases in the relative DNA copy number at those regions of the chromosome.

There are a number of variables in the CGH technique and analysis that are particularly important. For example, if the chromosomes are not correctly identified, the resultant profiles will be skewed and authentic deletions or amplifications may be missed (or alternatively, significant findings may be erroneously determined). If the hybridization is not fairly smooth and uniform across each metaphase or the illumination of the microscope is not even across the field, the intensity measurements will not be accurate. There are many reasons for each of these deficiencies, including uneven drying of the metaphase preparation, poor label incorporation in the probe, inefficient hybridization, chromatic abnormalities of the microscope, and an almost endless list of other variables that could affect the CGH outcome. CGH is an incredibly powerful screening tool, but its technical demands are not to be underestimated.

4. Notes

Clinical Applications: CGH was originally reported for the research-based analysis of solid tumors. Most of the publications to date continue to use CGH for this purpose with some success in identification of genetic deletions and amplifications important in various tumor types. Since its introduction, CGH has also been applied to leukemias and lymphomas, and a number of clinical applications have been suggested. In most clinical diagnostic situations, however, time is of the essence, and any diagnostic technique must produce results quickly, accurately, and reproducibly. For these reasons, CGH technology today may not be acceptable for many clinical applications. The following examples illustrate these limitations. CGH could theoretically be used to screen prenatal samples for trisomies and monosomies across the genome. The time required for the present CGH technology, however, makes this less useful than other FISH-based screening techniques using a combination of centromeric and single-copy probes for the clinically significant trisomies and monosomies *(13,18,21,X,Y)* that can be processed in the same day that the sample is collected. Because the hybridization kinetics of CGH do not allow for analysis at the telomeric and centromeric sequences, this technique is not useful for the identification of the chromosomes involved in cryptic, unbalanced translocations, which involve the telomeric sequences of one chromosome. The time required for CGH hybridization and analysis, as well as the requirement for a relatively large sample for DNA preparation, makes CGH less useful for analysis of small numbers of cells such as in preimplantation diagnostics. While the

DNA can be amplified using universal primers, the nonuniformity of the amplification remains a limitation. The second generation CGH technologies may overcome many of these limitations, but the technique will undoubtedly remain technically demanding. Even today, in the most experienced and skilled hands, CGH does not provide analyzable results in a significant proportion of the samples attempted.

References

1. Kallioniemi, A., Kallioniemi, O.-P., Sudar, D., Rutovitz, D., Gray, J. W., Waldman, F., and Pinkel, D. (1992) Comparative genomic hybridization for molecular cytogenetic analysis of solid tumors. *Science* **258,** 818–821.
2. Kallioniemi, A., Kallioniemi, O.-P., Piper, J., Tanner, M., Stokke, T., Chen, L., Smith, H. S., Pinkel, D., Gray, J. W., and Waldman, F. M. (1994) Detection and mapping of amplified DNA sequences in breast cancer by comparative genomic hybridization. *Proc. Natl. Acad. Sci. USA* **91,** 2156–2160.
3. Visakorpi, T., Kallioniemi, A. H., Syvanen, A.-C., Hyytinen, E. R., Karhu, R., Tammela, T., Isola, J. J., and Kallioniemi, O.-P. (1995) Genetic changes in primary and recurrent prostate cancer by comparative genomic hybridization. *Cancer Res.* **55,** 342–347.
4. Moch, H., Presti, Jr., J. C., Sauter, G., Buchholz, N., Jordan, P., Mihatsch, M. J., and Waldman, F. M. (1996) Genetic aberrations detected by comparative genomic hybridization are associated with clinical outcome in renal cell carcinoma. *Cancer Res.* **56,** 27–30.
5. Feuerstein, B. G. and Mohapatra, G. (1995) Molecular cytogenetic quantitation of gains and losses of genetic material from human gliomas. *J. Neurooncol.* **24(1),** 47–55.
6. Iwabuchi, H., Sakamoto, M., Sakunaga, H., Ma, Y. Y., Carcangiu, M. L., Pinkel, D., Yang-Feng, T. L., and Gray, J. W. (1995) Genetic analysis of benign, low-grade, and high-grade ovarian tumors. *Cancer Res.* **55,** 6172–6180.
7. Bentz, M., Dohner, H., Cabot, G., and Lichter, P. (1994) Fluorescence *in situ* hybridization in leukemias: "the FISH are spawning!" *Leukemia* **8(9),** 1447–1452.
8. Bryndorf, T., Kirchhoff, M., Rose, H., Maahr, J., Gerdes, T., Karhu, R., Kallioniemi, A., Christensen, B., Lundsteen, C., and Philip, J. (1995) Comparative genomic hybridization in clinical cytogenetics. *Am. J. Hum. Genet.* **57(5),** 1211–1220.
9. Speicher, M. R., du Manoir, S., Schrock, Holtgreve-Grez, H., Schoell, B., Lengauer, C., Cremer, T., and Ried, T. (1993) Molecular cytogenetic analysis of formalin-fixed, paraffin-embedded solid tumors by comparative genomic hybridization after universal DNA-amplification. *Hum. Mol. Genet.* **2(11),** 1907–1914.
10. Zhang, L., Cui, X., Schmitt, K., Hubert, R., Navidi, W., and Arnheim, N. (1992) Whole genome amplification from a single cell: implications for genetic analysis. *Proc. Natl. Acad. Sci. USA* **89,** 5847–5851.
11. Kallioniemi, O.-P., Kallioniemi, A., Piper, J., Isola, J., Waldman, F. M., Gray, J. W., and Pinkel, D. (1994) Optimizing comparative genomic hybridization for analysis of DNA sequence copy number changes in solid tumors. *Genes, Chromosomes & Cancer* **10,** 231–243.

12. Raap, T. (1995) Editorial: Comparative genomic hybridization. *Cytometry* **19**, 1–3.
13. du Manoir, S., Kallioniemi, O.-P., Lichter, P., Piper, J., Benedetti, P. A., Carothers, A. D., Fantes, J. A., Garcia-Sagredo, J. M., Gerdes, T., Giollant, M., Hemery, B., Isola, J., Maahr, J., Morrison, H., Perry, P., Stark, M., Sudar, D., van Vliet, L. J., Verwoerd, N., and Vrolijk, J. (1995) Hardware and software requirements for quantitative analysis of comparative genomic hybridization. *Cytometry* **19**, 4–9.
14. Piper, J., Rutovitz, D., Sudar, D., Kallioniemi, A., Kallioniemi, O.-P., Waldman, F. M., Gray, J. W., and Pinkel, D. (1995) Computer image analysis of comparative genomic hybridization. *Cytometry* **19**, 10–26.
15. du Manoir, S., Schrock, E., Bentz, M., Speicher, M. R., Joos, S., Ried, T., Lichter, P., and Cremer, T. (1995) Quantitative analysis of comparative genomic hybridization. *Cytometry* **19**, 27–41.
16. Lundsteen, C., Maahr, J., Christensen, B., Bryndorf, T., Bentz, M., Lichter, P., and Gerdes, T. (1995) Image analysis in comparative genomic hybridization. *Cytometry* **19**, 42–50.

15

In Situ Hybridization of Cells and Tissue Sections

Simon J. Conway

1. Introduction

In situ hybridization (ISH) has become a powerful and versatile method for the detection and localization of nucleic acid sequences within cells or tissue preparations. The technique provides a high degree of spatial information; specific DNA or RNA sequences can be located within a small subpopulation of cells, chromosomes or even individual cells within a tissue sample. ISH can be used to identify sites of gene expression, identify and localize viral infection, follow changes in specific mRNA synthesis, and map chromosomes.

Detecting messenger RNAs in individual cells and tissues has become a standard technique of molecular biology that is used in a broad range of disciplines from developmental biology to pathology *(1)*. The analysis of gene expression patterns can yield clues about the function(s) of the gene of interest. In addition to offering information about the normal tissue context of gene expression, ISH offers a potential advantage in sensitivity over filter hybridization in cases where the sequence of interest is present in only a small number of cells within a large mixed population. Such sequences may be undetectable in tissue extracts owing to dilution by other sequences from the surrounding tissue. The technique is especially powerful in the study of tissue, such as human and embryonic material, where RNA cannot easily be prepared from single tissues owing to the difficulty of dissection and the small amounts of material obtained. In contrast, ISH enables the localization of several different sequences with a single tissue sample or embryo. This technique is also complementary with tissue that has previously been prepared for histopathology.

The principle of the technique is simple. In brief, a single-stranded antisense probe of complementary sequence to the sense-strand RNA of interest, is hybridized to the sense RNA in a fixed tissue section. The remaining unbound

From: *Methods in Molecular Medicine, Molecular Diagnosis of Cancer*
Edited by: F. E. Cotter Humana Press Inc., Totowa, NJ

probe is then removed and the sites of hybridization are revealed, using autoradiography for radioactively-labeled probes and a "color reaction" detection method for nonradioactive probes. When adjacent sections are hybridized with antisense and sense RNA probes as a control, any signals seen only with the antisense probe can be assumed to be specific signals.

2. Materials

2.1. Preparation of Probes

1. Sterile distilled water treated with diethylpyrocarbonate (DEPC).
2. 10X Transcription buffer: 400 mM Tris-HCl, pH 8.25, 60 mM MgCl$_2$, 20 mM spermidine.
3. 0.2M DTT.
4. 2.5 mM GTP/ATP/CTP mix, pH 8.0.
5. Linearized plasmid (1 μg/μL).
6. Placental ribonuclease inhibitor (100 U/μL).
7. ^{35}S-UTP (1000–1500 Ci/mmol).
8. SP6, T7, or T3 RNA polymerase (10 U/μL).
9. Deoxyribonuclease I: 50 mg/mL—ribonuclease-free.
10. Alkaline hydrolysis solution: 0.2M NaHCO$_3$ and Na$_2$CO$_3$.
11. Yeast RNA (10 mg/mL).
12. Sephadex G50 or Biogel A1.5m column.
13. Column buffer: 10 mM Tris-HCl, 1 mM EDTA (pH 7.5), 10 mM DTT, 0.1% SDS.
14. 6M Ammonium acetate, pH 5.2.
15. Absolute ethanol.
16. 80% Ethanol.
17. Hybridization buffer: 50% deionized formamide, 0.3M NaCl, 20 mM Tris-HCl, 5 mM EDTA, pH 8.0, 10% dextran sulfate, 1X Denhardt's solution, 0.5 mg/mL yeast RNA. Store in aliquots at –70°C. Avoid freeze-thawing the probes.

2.2. Preparation of Slides and Coverslips

2.2.1. Slides

1. 10% HCl/70% ethanol.
2. Distilled water (DEPC-treated).
3. 95% Ethanol.
4. TESPA (3-aminopropyltriethoxysilane—Sigma number A3648): 2% in acetone.
5. Acetone.

2.2.2. Coverslips

1. 100% Ethanol.
2. Acetone.
3. Distilled water (DEPC-treated).

2.3. Tissue Fixation, Embedding and Sectioning

2.3.1. Wax Embedding

1. Phosphate buffered saline (PBS) treated with DEPC and sterilized by autoclaving.
2. Paraformaldehyde (4%) (PFA) in PBS (PFA 8 g in 180 mL sterile water is dissolved at 65°C on the day of use. Add five drops of 1*M* NaOH and cool to room temperature, then add 20 mL of 10X PBS). It is toxic and skin contact or inhalation should be avoided.
3. PBS:ethanol (1:1).
4. 50, 70, 85, 90, and 100% Ethanol.
5. Xylene, toluene, or Histoclear.
6. Histoclear:wax (1:1) (*see* Note 1).

2.3.2. Frozen Sections

1. Tissue-Tek OCT embedding medium.
2. Liquid nitrogen.
3. 4% Paraformaldehyde in PBS.
4. PBS.
5. 30, 50, 70, 85, 95, 99 and 100% Ethanol.

2.4. Prehybridization

1. Histoclear.
2. 100, 95, 85, 75, 50, and 30% Ethanol.
3. Saline (0.83% NaCl).
4. PBS.
5. Paraformaldehyde (4%) in PBS.
6. Proteinase K: 1 µg/mL, freshly diluted from 10 mg/mL stock in 50 m*M* Tris-HCl, 5 m*M* EDTA, pH 8.0. Buffer is sterilized by autoclaving.
7. Glycine: 2 mg/mL in PBS
8. Triethanolamine HCl: 0.1*M*, pH 8.0. Triethanolamine is sterilized by autoclaving.
9. Acetic anhydride (this is toxic and volatile).

2.5. Hybridization

1. Dithiothreitol (DTT).
2. Hybridization buffer (*see* Section 2.1.).
3. Tissue paper.
4. 50% Formamide.
5. 5X SSC: 0.3*M* NaCl, 0.03*M* trisodium citrate, pH 7.0.

2.6. Washing

1. Wash solution 1: 5X SSC and 10 m*M* DTT.
2. Wash solution 2: 50% formamide, 2X SSC, 10 m*M* DTT.
3. Wash solution 3: NTE buffer consisting of 0.5*M* NaCl, 10 m*M* Tris-HCl, 5 m*M* EDTA, pH 8.0.

4. Wash solution 4: 20 μg/mL ribonuclease A in NTE buffer.
5. Wash solution 5: 2X SSC.
6. Wash solution 6: 0.1X SSC.
7. 30, 60, 80, and 95% Ethanol (ethanol dilutions made with distilled water containing 0.3*M* ammonium acetate).
8. 100% Ethanol.

2.7. Preliminary Autoradiographic Check

1. Autoradiographic film (Beta Max–Hyperfilm).
2. 3MM paper.

2.8. Autoradiography

1. Kodak Wratten series II safelight.
2. Water bath set at 45°C.
3. Large light-tight box.

2.8.1. Preparation

1. Autoradiographic emulsion (Ilford K5) (prediluted vials of emulsion, stored at 4°C) diluted 1:1 with distilled water containing 600 m*M* sodium acetate, giving a final concentration of 300 m*M* and 1% glycerol to prevent cracking.
2. Sterile water.
3. Desiccant beads.
4. Aluminium foil.

2.8.2. Development of Slides

Make up fresh reagents:

1. Developer: Ilford Phenisol 1:4 solution.
2. Stop bath: 2–5 drops acetic acid in cold sterile water.
3. Fixer: 30% sodium thiosulfate or a commercial fixer (e.g., Ilford Rapid fix).

2.8.3. Staining

1. Staining solution (0.02% toluidine blue/water).
2. Distilled water.
3. 70, 100% Ethanol.
4. Xylene.

3. Methods

3.1. Preparation of Probes

Radioactive and nonradioactive probes can be synthesized in a number of ways. Kits can be brought to make random primed or end labeled double-stranded DNA probes, or single-stranded RNA probes. Generally, single-stranded antisense RNA probes are preferred to double-stranded DNA probes, as single-stranded RNA probes have been shown to be more sensitive—up to eight times that achieved with double-stranded DNA probes *(2)* and give more reproducible results. Antisense RNA probes offer several advantages. First, and most importantly, is the ability to use ribonuclease to reduce nonspecific background as RNA/RNA duplexes are resistant to mild RNase treatment. Second, there is no complementary sense strand to compete for probe in the hybridization as there would be with a double-stranded DNA probe. Third, a higher wash temperature can be used, as the binding between RNA/RNA duplexes is stronger than between RNA/DNA duplexes. Also, DNA probes offer no sense/antisense comparison, so having good controls may be a problem.

However, DNA oligonucleotides can be useful for certain studies, as it is possible to design probes that distinguish transcripts with a few sequence differences, e.g., closely related members of a gene family or alternatively spliced RNAs from the same gene. A problem with the use of oligonucleotides is that they are relatively insensitive owing to their low complexity, but probes as short as 25 bases have been shown to give specific hybridization when target abundance is high *(3)*, although longer probes show increased hybridization signals.

The choice of label depends on the resolution required. Low-energy 3H probes allow accurate localization of the target sequence within a single cell and are both cheap and last for a long time. However, owing to the low specific activity of 3H, long exposures of weeks or even months are required to achieve a satisfactory detectable signal. Therefore, ^{35}S-labeled probes are more commonly used: they can be synthesized to a high specific-activity and give good cellular resolution relatively rapidly, and last for 6–8 wk. When using DNA probes, high specific-activity ^{32}P-labeled probes can be used and give immediate results, but the resolution is poor and the probes have to be used quickly before they degrade (within a couple of days). Nonradioactive techniques for ISH and whole-mount ISH have also been developed. Whole-mount ISH offers several advantages: particularly simplification of the detection and interpretation of gene expression patterns, rapid results, indefinite storage of probes, and, most importantly, safety *(4,5)*. Nevertheless, these methods are at present less sensitive than radioactive probes, and are not compatible with other routine histopathology procedures.

3.2. Preparation of ^{35}S-Radiolabeled Probe

Single-stranded RNA probes are synthesized by in vitro transcription with high efficiency, and thus high specific activity from either the T3, T7, or Sp6 RNA polymerase bacterial promoters. Several vectors such as Bluescript, Bluescribe, pGEM, or SP6 plasmid vectors are useful *(6)*. In order to transcribe the insert and not the plasmid, the vector must be linearized with an enzyme that cleaves downstream of the insert in the multiple cloning site. The digest is then phenol-extracted, washed with ethanol, dried, and redissolved in sterile distilled water. Details of subcloning, linearization, and isolation of plasmid DNA can be obtained from ref. 7.

The transcription reaction and all subsequent reactions must be free of ribonuclease (*see* Note 3). Three unlabeled and one radioactive ribonucleotide are used to transcribe the probe. UTP is the ribonucleotide of choice as the polymerase enzymes have the highest affinity for this nucleotide, and, as such, probes of high specific activity can be synthesized. Very high specific-activity probes can also be synthesized using two unlabeled and two radioactive ribonucleotides. The amount of probe synthesized can be determined from the incorporation in disintegrations/min and the specific activity of the isotope (Ci/mmol) by using the following formula:

$$\text{RNA synthesized (ng)} = (\text{dpm} \times 9.1 \times 10-4) / \text{Ci/mmol}$$

The incorporation is usually between 50 and 80%. A good reaction will yield 1 mg of probe with a specific activity of $6\text{--}8 \times 10^8$ dpm./μg of probe.

It has been found that the optimal length of probe is around 100 bases, presumably enabling easy tissue penetration. Thus, if large inserts are transcribed, the RNA can be reduced in size by limited alkaline hydrolysis, as described in steps 5 and 6 of the following protocol. However, it is best to use an insert of around 100–200 bases, and avoid alkaline hydrolysis—as sometimes this results in high backgrounds. In practice, transcription usually results in the majority of the transcripts of the RNA probe being less than full length.

3.2.1. Synthesis of Single-Stranded RNA Probes

1. Mix the following reagents in the order at room temperature: 3 μL sterile distilled water, 2 μL 10X transcription buffer, 1 μL 0.2M DTT, 2 μL 2.5 mM GTP/ATP/CTP mix, 1 μL linearized plasmid, 0.5 μL placental ribonuclease inhibitor, 10 μL ^{35}S-UTP, and 0.5 μL SP6, T7, or T3 RNA polymerase.
2. Incubate at 37°C for 1 h.
3. Add 50 mg/mL deoxyribonuclease I to remove DNA template.
4. Incubate at 37°C for 15 min.
5. Add an equal volume (20 μL) of alkaline hydrolysis solution.
6. Reduce probe size to 100 bases by incubating at 60°C for *t* min, where:

$$t = (\text{Lo} - \text{Lf})/(0.11 \times \text{Lo} \times \text{Lf})$$

(Lo is the original probe length and Lf is the desired probe length in kb).
7. Add 1 μL of yeast RNA.
8. Separate RNA from unincorporated nucleotides by fractionation on a Sephadex G50 or Biogel A1.5m column (e.g., in a Pasteur pipet) using column buffer. Determine the radioactivity present in an aliquot of each fraction; the first peak eluted will contain the probe and the second peak will consist of unincorporated nucleotides.

9. Pool the peak fractions containing probe, add 0.5 vol of 6*M* ammonium acetate, 2 vol of ethanol and incubate at –20°C for a minimum of 2 h or at –70°C for 30 min.
10. Centrifuge at 13,000*g* for 20 min and wash pellet in 80%, then 100% ethanol before drying.
11. Resuspend pellet at 2×10^6 cpm/µL in 100 m*M* DTT.
12. Add 9 vol of hybridization buffer and store at –70°C.

3.3. Slide and Coverslip Preparation

Tissue sections or cells undergo a variety of relatively harsh treatments during the hybridization and washing steps. Hence, the slides should be thoroughly cleaned, sterilized, and coated to facilitate tissue adhesion. Slides can be stored dust-free at room temperature and used several months after coating.

3.3.1. Slides

1. Dip slides in 10% HCl/70% ethanol, followed by distilled water, and then 95% ethanol.
2. Dry in oven at 150°C for 5 min and allow to cool.
3. Dip slides in 2% TESPA in acetone for 10 s.
4. Wash twice with acetone and then distilled water (DEPC-treated).
5. Dry at 42°C.

3.3.2. Coverslips

1. Wash in acetone and store in beaker of 100% ethanol.
2. Wash twice in 100% ethanol and dry for 10 min.
3. Immerse in silane for 2 min and dry.
4. Wash twice in water (DEPC-treated).

3.4. Tissue Fixation, Embedding, and Sectioning

Fixation is one of the most important steps in obtaining good ISH results. Optimal fixation and sample penetration must retain the maximal level of cellular target RNA while maintaining morphology and allowing access of the probe. There are two methods commonly used for the preparation of tissue for ISH. Samples can either be frozen in liquid nitrogen and sectioned on a cryostat, or fixed with a crosslinking fixative and embedded in paraffin wax prior to sectioning. Messenger RNA is enzymatically degraded by RNases, thus tissue should be fixed or frozen as soon as possible for optimal results—within 10 min of tissue extraction is a safe limit. Tissues are kept on ice during preparation before fixation, so as to reduce the effects of RNase. Cryostat sectioning requires less tissue preparation, and may be more sensitive, but the sectioning of wax-embedded tissue is the most commonly used

method. Wax sections yield better tissue preservation, allow serial sectioning, and can be stored almost indefinitely. Fixation in paraformaldehyde, followed by embedding in wax, is the best compromise allowing permeability
and good target retention.

3.4.1. Wax Embedding

1. Dissect out tissue in ice-cold PBS.
2. Place in ice-cold 4% PFA in PBS and leave at 4°C overnight.
3. Successively replace solution with the following, each for at least 30 min and
   with occasional agitation: PBS at 4°C twice; PBS:ethanol (1:1); 50% ethanol;
   and 70, 85, 90, and 100% ethanol. Absolute (100%) ethanol must be used for the
   efficient penetration of wax. For large samples, these times must be increased.
   Samples can be stored indefinitely in any of the alcohol solutions.
4. Replace solution with xylene, Toluene, or Histoclear, twice for 1 h each, then a
   Histoclear:wax (1:1) mix at 60°C for 30 min, followed by three changes of wax,
   each for 40 min. It is important not to exceed these times, unless this is necessary
   for larger samples, such as adult tissues.
5. Transfer samples to a mould, orientate, and allow to set. For convenience,
   use glass embryological dishes (Raymond Lamb) placed on a heater block at
   60°C. The samples can be orientated under a dissecting microscope using a
   warmed needle.
6. Store at 4°C until required for sectioning.
7. Cut ribbons of 5–10 μm sections.
8. When required part of tissue is reached, place sections onto a subbed slide containing a large drop of water on a hotplate at 45°C.
9. Float sections until creases disappear: the section should expand to its original size.
10. Dry slides at 37°C overnight and store desiccated at 4°C.

3.4.2. Frozen Sections

1. Place tissue in tin foil mould half filled with OCT embedding medium.
2. Fill mould with OCT.
3. Touch mould onto surface of liquid nitrogen until solid.
4. Store at –70°C . Blocks frozen for 3 mo can give good results.
5. Remove blocks from –70 to –20°C and trim with razor blade, mount onto cryostat
   chuck using OCT and rapid cooling on dry ice.
6. Cut sections at –20°C at 8–10 μm.
7. When required part reached, pick up individual sections by slowly bringing
   subbed slide at room temperature next to section.
8. Air dry sections onto slides for a few minutes at room temperature—dust free.
9. Fix in 4% PFA in PBS for 20 min.
10. Wash 2 × 5 min in PBS.
11. Dehydrate in ethanol series: 30 s each in 30, 50, 70, 85, 95, 99, and 100% water.
12. Air dry for 10 min.
13. Store as wax sections.

3.5. Prehybridization

A number of prehybridization treatments are used to improve signal and reduce nonspecific binding during hybridization (background). Paraffin sections require dewaxing, then rehydration. The tissue is then permeablized by proteinase K digestion of protein to allow entry of the probe. The protease is inhibited using glycine, and an acetylation step is used to help reduce background by blocking amino residues. Postfixation enables the morphology to be maintained.

1. Dewax slides in Histoclear, twice for 10 min, and then place in 100% ethanol for 2 min to remove most of the xylene.
2. Transfer slides quickly (30 s) through 100% ethanol (twice), 95, 85, 75, 50, and then 30% ethanol.
3. Transfer slides to saline, and then PBS for 5 min each.
4. Immerse slides in fresh 4% paraformaldehyde in PBS for 20 min.
5. Wash with PBS, twice for 5 min.
6. Drain slides, place them in a dish containing 1 μg/mL proteinase K. Leave for 30 min at 37°C.
7. Place in 2 mg/mL glycine in PBS for 30 s to block the proteinase reaction.
8. Wash with PBS for 5 min.
9. Repeat fixation in 4% paraformaldehyde in PBS for 20 min. The same solution from step 4 can be used.
10. Wash in distilled water and place in $0.1M$ triethanolamine HCl set up with a rapidly rotating stir bar, in a fume hood.
11. Add 1/400 of acetic anhydride and leave for 10 min.
12. Wash with PBS and then saline for 5 min each.
13. Dehydrate slides quickly passing through 30, 50, 70, 85, 95, and 100% ethanol twice. To avoid salt deposits on the slides, they should be left in 70% ethanol for 5 min.
14. Air-dry and use on the same day for hybridization.

3.6. Hybridization and Washing Sections

Hybridization of the probe to the target RNA is usually complete after 4–6 h, but for convenience, hybridization is carried out overnight *(8)*. The optimum probe concentration is that which gives the best signal-to-noise ratio. This is the concentration that just saturates the target RNAs: the formula is 0.3 μg/mL of probe per kb of probe length (*see* ref. *2*). However, for convenience, probes are used at a concentration of 300 ng/mL in the hybridization buffer. Before hybridization, the probes are heat denatured in order to remove any possible secondary structure that would inhibit hybridization. Always keep the probe in a reduced state by adding DTT, as this helps to keep the background minimal.

3.6.1. Hybridization

1. Heat hybridization mix including probe at 80°C for 2 min (*see* Section 3.2.1., step 12).
2. Vortex and spin probe to mix and remove any bubbles.
3. Apply hybridization mix to slide, adjacent to sections. Approximately 10 μL/18 × 18-mm slide (15 μL for large tissues).
4. Gently lower a clean coverslip so that the hybridization mix is spread over the sections.
5. Place slides horizontally in a plastic slide box, together with tissue paper soaked in 50% formamide, 5X SSC, and seal the box to form a moist chamber. The box is arranged in the oven such that the slides have the sections facing up, with the coverslips on top.
6. Incubate overnight at 50–55°C.

3.6.2. Washing

It is important to keep the tissues moist, therefore transfer the slides into racks already immersed in solutions whenever possible. DTT is labile, and thus is the last item added to solutions. It is important to remove the formaldehyde and DTT completely before the RNase step, otherwise the RNase is inactivated. The RNase A step should eliminate nonspecific hybridization, as bonafide hybrids are RNase resistant.

1. Remove slides and place in a slide rack in wash solution 1 at 50°C for 30–60 min for coverslips to fall off.
2. Place slides in wash solution 2 either at 50°C for 60 min for low-stringency washing or at 65°C for 30 min for high-stringency washing.
3. Wash three times for 10 min each with wash solution 3 at 37°C.
4. Treat with wash solution 4 at 37°C for 30 min.
5. Wash with wash solution 3 at 37°C for 15 min.
6. Repeat either the low or high-stringency wash of step 2.
7. Wash in wash solution 5, and then wash solution 6 for 15 min each at 37°C.
8. Dehydrate slides by quickly putting them through 30, 60, 80, and 95% ethanol (including ammonium acetate), followed by 100% ethanol, twice.
9. Air-dry for 30 min, then use for autoradiography.

3.7. Preliminary Autoradiographic Check

Rather than dipping the slides and developing test slides over a time period, the slides can be placed against an autoradiographic film (Beta Max – Hyperfilm) to produce a low-resolution image. Using a rough relationship that a 1-d exposure on Beta Max equals a 3-d exposure of dipped slides, it is possible to get a rough idea of how long to expose the dipped slides for. This step can also be used to test whether the experiment has worked, and so whether it is worthwhile to proceed to dip and expose the slides. An example of exposure to auto-radiographic film can be seen in Fig. 1A.

1. Place slides on 3MM paper and stick down with tape, section side up.
2. Place slides against autoradiographic film under safelight conditions.
3. Develop 24 h later and check background vs signal. If there is no difference, then put against an autoradiograph for 48 h.

3.8. Autoradiography

All of these steps are carried out in the darkroom. The autoradiographic emulsion is very sensitive to light. All the following steps are to be carried out under safelight conditions (Kodak Wratten series II safelight). The darkroom should be equipped with a water bath set at 45°C, a dipping chamber, and a large light-tight box to dry the emulsion after application to the slides (*see* Note 4).

3.8.1. Preparation

1. Set water bath at 45°C.
2. Use prediluted vials of emulsion (stored at 4°C), which are diluted 1:1 with distilled water containing 600 m*M* sodium acetate, giving a final concentration of 300 m*M* and 1% glycerol to prevent cracking.
3. Boil slide chamber (10 mL vol) in sterile water to clean.
4. Unwrap emulsion vial (stored in 10-mL aliquots) and leave in water bath for 20 min to melt.
5. Fill chamber with emulsion.
6. Check emulsion is bubble free by dipping a clean slide and examining it for an even coating. Repeat this until bubbles are removed. Next, dip the experimental slides, allowing each to drain vertically for 2 s, wiping the back of the slide and placing it vertically in a wooden rack to dry.
7. Transfer all slides to plastic tray and dry for 1 h. It is important that the slides are completely dry during exposure.
8. Place tray in a glass dish with desiccant beads in the bottom, covered with paper towel. A lump of tape can be stuck on the front right hand side of the dish so as to locate the position of the tray in the dark.
9. Wrap dish in three sheets of new foil and place at 4°C.
10. The refrigerator used must not be used to store radioactive sources. In addition, the emulsion is sensitive to shock, so the slides must be treated gently.
11. Exposure times can be calculated approximately from the preliminary autoradiographic test (*see* Note 5).

3.8.2. Development of Slides

1. Remove box of slides from 4°C and warm to room temperature (1–2 h).
2. Under safelight conditions, using a Kodak Wratten series II safelight, in a darkroom, transfer the slides through developer to fix.

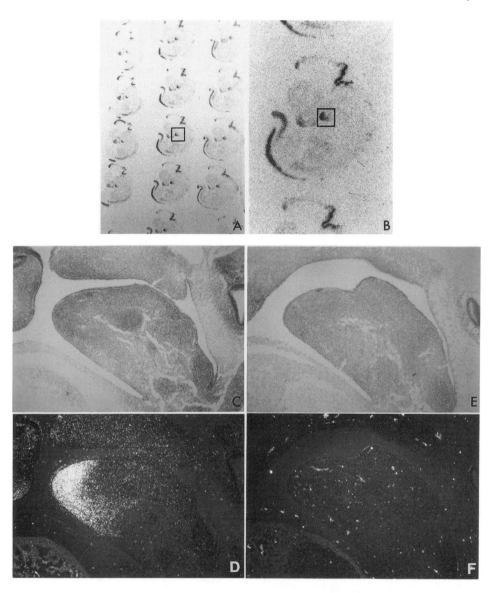

Fig. 1. Hybridization of ^{35}S-labeled Pax3 mouse sense and antisense probes to mouse sections. Sagittal sections through a 13-d-old embryo reveal Pax3 mRNA expression in the neural tube, mid- and hind-brain, and upper and lower jaws. High-stringency washes were carried out to obtain low nonspecific background. (A–D) were hybridized with the antisense probe, and (E) and (F) were hybridized with the control sense probe. **(A)** Light-field photograph of the exposure left on the autoradiographic film after 4 d. Several consecutive sections all display the same expression patterns. **(B)** Enlargement of A. **(C)** Light-field photograph of the dipped and exposed slide

3. Make up fresh reagents:
   a. Developer: Ilford Phenisol 1:4 solution for 5 min at 19°C.
   b. Stop bath: 2–5 drops acetic acid in cold sterile water.
   c. Fixer: 30% sodium thiosulfate or a commercial fixer (e.g., Ilford Rapid fix) for 5 min.
   (The temperature of the developer is critical, as it effects the size of the silver grains produced; the warmer the developer, the larger the grains).
4. Wash in tap water for 10 min. The light can now be turned on.

3.8.3. Staining

1. Stain lightly in a 0.02% Toluidine blue/water staining solution.
2. Wash the slides twice in distilled water for 10 min, quickly transfer through 70 and 100% ethanol, xylene twice, and air-dry.
3. Add the coverslip and lay slides flat overnight to dry.

3.9. Photography

The localization of silver grains can be seen under both bright-field and dark-field illumination, but dark-field allows more accurate visualization. This can be seen in Fig. 1.

4. Notes

1. Many alternative paraffin waxes can be used, such as pastillated Fibrowax (BDH).
2. "3' overhang enzymes" 'hang on' and start to reverse transcribe the opposite strand. If you are forced to use a 3' overhang, then the digest should be blunt-ended (e.g., T4).
3. It is essential to bake (180°C) or autoclave all tubes and pipet tips. Double-distilled water used for all buffers (except Tris and EDTA, which inactivate DEPC) should be treated with 0.1% DEPC and sterilized by autoclaving. Gloves should be worn at all times to avoid contamination with ribonucleases.
4. The autographic emulsion has a gelatin base. It is solid at room temperature and becomes liquid at 45°C.
5. The following are various problems that can be encountered together with some possible causes and appropriate remedies:
   a. Low hybridization signal
   • A low probe concentration, which can be remedied by increasing the probe concentration. The amount of probe should be checked after purification.
   • Degradation by nuclease digestion. Ensure all appropriate solutions and equipment are sterilized, this is particularly important for RNA probes and target RNA. Wear gloves at all times.

---

after 12 d. A magnified image of the Pax3 mRNA expression in the lower jaw is shown. **(D)** Dark-field photograph of C. **(E)** Light-field photograph of the lower jaw is shown. There is no hybridization with the sense probe. **(F)** Dark-field photograph of E. Magnifications: A ×40; B ×100; C–F ×400.

- Large probe size. Alkaline hydrolysis to reduce probe size (RNA probes). Optimize hydrolysis time for each of the RNA probes.
- Poor probe labeling: the label incorporation should be checked. Ensure the use of control reagents for labeling reaction.
- Low specific activity: can be altered by using fresh radioactive label.
- Short autoradiography exposure, which can be changed by increasing exposure time (check exposure with film first).

b. High background:

- Long autoradiography exposure, which can be changed by decreasing exposure time (check exposure with film first).
- Emulsion—use fresh emulsion and developing chemicals.
- High probe concentration (check probe amount after purification)—reduce probe concentration.
- Emulsion exposed to light/radiation before or during exposure check light tightness of darkroom and storage conditions.
- Patchy background signal. Check emulsion—clean all old emulsion from dipping chamber before reuse.

References

1. Harris, N. and Wilkinson, D. (eds.) (1990) *In Situ Hybridisation: Application to Development Biology and Medicine*, Cambridge University Press, Cambridge, UK.
2. Cox, K. H., DeLeon, D. V., Angerer, L. M., and Angerer, R. C. (1984) Detection of mRNA's in Sea Urchin embryos by *in situ* hybridisation using asymmetric RNA probes. *Dev. Biol.* **101**, 485–502.
3. Berger, C. N. (1986) *In situ* hybridisation of immunoglobulin-specific RNA in single cells of the B lymphocyte lineage with radiolabelled DNA probes. *EMBO J.* **5**, 85–93.
4. Rosen, B. and Beddington, R. S. (1993) Whole-mount *in situ* hybridisation in the mouse embryo: gene expression in three dimensions. *Trends Genet.* **9**, 162–167.
5. Strähle, U., Bladder, P., Adam, J., and Ingham, P. W. (1994) A simple and efficient procedure for non-isotopic *in situ* hybridisation to sectioned material. *Trends Genet.* **10**, 75,76.
6. Melton, D. A., Krieg, P. A., Rebagliati, M. R., Maniatis, T., Zinn, K., and Green, M. R. (1984) Efficient in vitro synthesis of biologically active RNA and RNA hybridisation probes from plasmids containing a bacteriophage SP6 promoter. *Nucleic Acids Res.* **12**, 7035–7056.
7. Maniatis, T., Fritsch, E. F., and Sambrook, J. (eds.) (1982) *Molecular Cloning: A Laboratory Manual*, Cold Spring Harbor Laboratory, Cold Spring Harbor, NY.
8. Wilkinson, D. G. (ed.) (1992) *In Situ Hybridisation: A Practical Approach*, IRL Press, Oxford, UK.

16

Apoptosis Detection by DNA Analysis

Paul D. Allen and Adrian C. Newland

1. Introduction

Apoptosis is a series of controlled sequential events resulting in cell death. This complements proliferation in the maintenance of tissue homeostasis. The process is regulated to give a "shrinking cell" with a characteristic appearance. Apoptotic cells undergo compaction of nuclear chromatin and cytoplasmic condensation followed by budding of the cell to form membrane bound apoptotic bodies *(1,2)*. These contain varying proportions of cellular organelles and nuclear material and are rapidly phagocytosed by surrounding cells. Cell loss, therefore, is achieved without the induction of inflammation. The discovery that certain proto-oncogenes *(3)*, e.g., *c-myc* and *bcl*-2 and the tumor suppressor gene *p53* are implicated in the control of apoptosis has focused attention on both the role of apoptosis in tumorogenesis and as a possible pathway to which cancer therapeutic regimens could be directed *(4)*. The latter point is clinically relevant in that radiotherapy, hormone therapy, and a broad spectrum of chemotherapeutic agents all induce apoptotic death in target cells. Therefore, tumor resistance to these agents may well be associated with blockades or lesions in the apoptotic pathway.

Biochemically, apoptosis has been traditionally associated with the activation of an endonuclease activity causing double-stranded cleavage of DNA at internucleosomal sites. The result is fragmentation of DNA into multiples of 180 bp lengths *(5)*. A characteristic "ladder" effect is obtained when these fragments are resolved by agarose gel electrophoresis. DNA degradation of this type is usually found in cells that are morphologically apoptotic and the generation of "ladders" has been extensively used to define apoptosis in many experimental systems. However, DNA cleavage to this extent, is thought to represent an advanced stage of DNA fragmentation and the notion that DNA ladders are definitive for apoptosis no longer holds true.

From: *Methods in Molecular Medicine, Molecular Diagnosis of Cancer*
Edited by: F. E. Cotter Humana Press Inc., Totowa, NJ

Pulsed field gel electrophoresis (PFGE), has made it possible to separate and analyze large DNA fragments that could not have been resolved by conventional constant field electrophoresis. Numerous variations have been developed since PFGE was first described in 1983 and it has now been refined to analyze DNA fragments of over 10 Mbp. There are two main electrode configurations used in PFGE. One applies alternate transverse fields in two directions. Electrode configuration and reorientation angles differ depending whether orthogonal field electrophoresis (OFAGE), contour-clamped homogenous electric field (CHEF), or rotating field gel electrophoresis (ROFE) is used. The other electrode configuration is a one-dimensional reorientation process where the electrical field is reversed and is therefore known as field inversion gel electrophoresis (FIGE). Forward DNA migration is achieved by longer or greater field strengths in the forward direction than in the reversed direction. Apoptotic DNA is resolved using FIGE. Temporal studies on the induction of apoptosis in epithelial cell lines using FIGE analysis, have shown that internucleosomal cleavage of DNA into 180 bp multimers is preceded by the appearance of larger DNA fragments of 300 kbp and/or 50 kbp *(6,7)*. Moreover, in a cell line exhibiting 50 kbp fragmentation, no further degradation to 180 bp multimers was detected. It is now thought that large DNA fragmentation occurs before the subsequent degradation of DNA to oligonucleosomes lengths and that in some cells, at least, this final degradation process may not even take place. Therefore, the failure to resolve DNA into the classical ladders of apoptosis does not necessarily mean that the cells are not undergoing apoptosis and FIGE should be carried out to see whether larger DNA fragmentation into high molecular weight fragments has taken place.

2. Materials

1. Lysis buffer: 10 mM EDTA, 50 mM Tris-HCl, pH 8.0, 0.5% w/v N-lauroyl-sarcosine, and 0.5 mg/mL proteinase K. (Proteinase K is stored at –20°C and added separately when required.)
2. TE buffer: 10 mM Tris-HCl, pH 8.0 and 1 mM EDTA.
3. Tris/EDTA/NaCl buffer: 10 mM, Tris-HCl, pH 7.6, 100 mM, EDTA, and 20 mM sodium chloride.
4. Sample buffer: 10 mM EDTA, 0.25% w/v bromophenol blue, and 50% v/v glycerol.
5. TBE electrophoresis buffer: 2 mM EDTA, 89 mM Tris-HCl, pH 8.0, and 89 mM boric acid.
6. Tris-buffered phenol/chloroform: Melt the phenol in a water bath at 56°C and remove 20 mL. Sequentially add small volumes of 0.1M Tris-HCl, pH 7.4 to the phenol and constantly agitate the mix until the phenol also acquires a pH of 7.4. Allow the mix to separate and add phenol from the lower phase to an equal volume of chloroform just prior to use.
7. Chloroform isoamyl alcohol: Add 24 vol of chloroform to 1 vol of isoamyl alcohol just prior to use.

It is good practice to use sterile disposable plasticware in the preparation of reagents and in the isolation of the DNA. Pipet tips and Eppendorf tubes should be autoclaved if not purchased sterile. Sterile, distilled deionized water should be used for making up buffers and use molecular biology grade materials throughout. Particular care should be taken handling phenol and the organic solvents; a fume cupboard should be used where necessary. High molecular weight DNA fragmentation can be caused by DNase activity. Therefore, when isolating the DNA for FIGE, particular attention should be paid toward preventing contamination of materials and reagents with DNA nucleases. Wear gloves and use only sterile plastic and glassware. Do not use metal implements at any stage in the process.

3. Methods

3.1. Conventional Constant Field Gel Electrophoresis

1. Harvest apoptotic cells from culture and wash once in Hanks Balanced Salt Solution (HBSS).
2. Lyse cells at 1×10^7/mL in lysis buffer in an Eppendorf tube, e.g., 2×10^6 cells in 200 µL lysis buffer, and incubate for 1 h at 56°C in a waterbath.
3. Add ribonuclease A (RNase Type III-A) to a final concentration of 0.25 mg/mL. Incubate for a further 1 h at 56°C. Heat inactivate (80°C for 30 min) the RNase to denature any contaminating DNase activity.
4. Add 1 vol of a 1:1 mix of Tris buffered phenol and chloroform.
5. Mix thoroughly for 5 min by repeated inversion and centrifuge for 4 min at 800g in a bench top microfuge. Remove the lower organic layer *carefully* and discard.
6. Repeat steps 4 and 5.
7. Add 1 vol of a 24:1 mix of chloroform and isoamyl alcohol.
8. Mix thoroughly for 5 min by repeated inversion and centrifuge for 4 min at 800g in a bench top microfuge.
9. Carefully remove the majority of the upper aqueous phase and put into a fresh clean Eppendorf tube. *Avoid drawing up any of the organic phase.*
10. Add 1.5 vol of TE buffer.
11. Centrifuge at 13,000g for 10 min and collect the supernatant (which contains fragmented apoptotic DNA).
12. Add 2 vol of cold (4°C) 100% ethanol.
13. Mix by repeated inversion until DNA is precipitated (approx 20 min). The DNA can be stored overnight at this stage at −20°C.
14. Pellet the DNA by centrifugation at 13,000g for 10 min.
15. Discard the supernatant and allow the DNA pellet to dry (about 15 min).
16. Dissolve the DNA pellet in TE buffer (DNA from 2×10^6 cells will dissolved in 20 µL buffer).
17. Add 1 vol of sample buffer to 4 vol of DNA preparation. Aim to get 1–5 µg/mL DNA per well.
18. Load sample onto a submarine horizontal 1% agarose gel and electrophorese at 6 V/cm using 0.5% TBE running buffer. This takes approx 2 h on an 8-cm "mini" gel.

19. Stain gel in 1 μg/mL ethidium bromide (made up in running buffer) for 10 min and destain in running buffer or water until the background is clear.
20. Visualize on a UV transilluminator (*see* Note 1).
21. Gel can be photographed using a Polaroid DS 34 direct screen instant camera mounted on a DS H-8 0.8X hood.

3.2. Field Inversion Gel Electrophoresis (FIGE)

1. Harvest apoptotic cells and wash once in HBSS.
2. Resuspend 4×10^6 cells in 50 μL Tris/EDTA/NaCl buffer prewarmed to 37°C.
3. Add an equal volume 1.5% low melting point agarose. The agarose is melted in a microwave oven and allowed to cool to about 37°C
4. Mix gently, pour into the mold (*see the following*) and allow a plug to form on ice for 10 min.
5. Transfer the plug to a 1-mL vol of Tris/EDTA/NaCl buffer containing 1% lauroyl sarcosine and 1.0 mg/mL proteinase K.
6. Incubate overnight at 37°C (Plugs can be stored in 500 m*M* EDTA at 4°C at this stage).
7. Wash the plugs twice by rinsing them for 1 h in Tris/EDTA/NaCl buffer.
8. Cut plugs to contain 1–5 μg DNA and seal into a 1.5% agarose gel with 1% low melting point agarose (4×10^6 cells will yield approx 20–30 μg/mL of DNA) (*see* Note 2).
9. Subject the gel plugs to FIGE in a cold room (*see* Note 2). Electrophoresis is carried out in 0.5% TBE running buffer. Complete systems for PFGE are now commercially available consisting of power supply, pulse controller, electrophoresis unit containing built-in cooling systems, and electrode arrangements. Gel casting trays are also provided. However, FIGE can be carried out using standard power supply and gel electrophoresis apparatus so long as access can be gained to a suitable pulse controller with field inversion and a ramped range of pulse times. Several pulse controllers are commercially available. FIGE for resolution of large molecular weight apoptotic DNA fragments is started by an initial continuous forward pulse of 100 V for 15 min. Electrophoresis is then carried out at around 10 V/cm, i.e., 200 V for a gel run of 20 cm. A forward to backward ratio of 3:1 should be selected (forward pulse is three times longer than the reverse pulse). DNA fragments of 10 kbp to 1 Mbp can be resolved using a pulse ramping rate changing from 0.5 s to 10 s for 19 h, followed by 10 s to 60 s over the next 19 h. Also, a ramp from 1 s to 60 s over a 22-h period could be used. A shorter alternative protocol starts with a 15-min continuous forward pulse followed by a 2.4-s forward pulse and a 0.8-s reverse pulse (3:1 ratio again) for 1 h. This is then followed by a ramping rate changing up to 24 s forward (and 8 s reverse) over a run of 7 h. The field strengths stated above should be used (*see* Note 2).
10. Stain gels in 1 μg/mL ethidium bromide (made up in running buffer) for 10 min and destain in running buffer or water until the background is clear.
11. Gel can be photographed using a Polaroid DS 34 direct screen instant camera mounted on a DS H-8 0.8X hood (*see* Fig. 1).

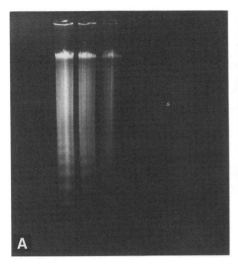
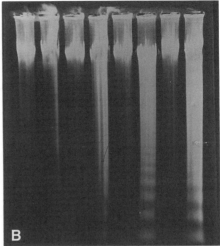

Fig. 1. (A) Oligonucleosomal length DNA fragments isolated from HL-60 cells irradiated by UV light on a transilluminator for 10 min and incubated for a further 2 h. DNA was resolved on a 1% agarose 8 cm "mini" gel using conventional constant field (6 V/cm) gel electrophoresis. **(B)** Oligonucleosomal length DNA fragments isolated from cells incubated with increasing concentrations of etoposide (lanes 2, 4, 6, and 8). Poor resolution of the ladder in lane 8 is symptomatic of lane overloading. Same conditions as for panel A.

4. Notes

1. Conventional Electrophoresis: Failure to resolve oligonucleosome lengths of DNA into ladders using conventional constant field electrophoresis could be owing to excessive loading of DNA, which gives a thick smear down the gel, and therefore should be reduced accordingly. The percentage agarose in the gels can also be increased anywhere up to 2%. Agarose gels of 1.8% have been reported in the literature. Greater resolution of bands also may be achieved by heating the final DNA preparation in sample buffer to 65°C and then rapidly cooling it on ice. The samples are then loaded onto the gel. Ladders easily can be seen using "mini" gels (8 cm), but again better resolution of bands can be obtained if longer gel runs are used (>14 cm). Finally, although DNA can be stored overnight or longer at stage 13 in the protocol, it is better to isolate the DNA and run the gel on the same day.

2. Field Inversion Electrophoresis: The technique of isolating DNA in agarose plugs was developed to prevent artificial cleavage of DNA during preparative procedures. Commercially available systems for PFGE come complete with insert molds that produce plugs of the correct size for loading into the wells of the resolving gel. However, molds can be made by a variety of techniques. When designing the mold, the total yield of DNA must be borne in mind and whether

the plug size that can be obtained from the mold will contain in the order of 1–5 µg DNA. The method outlined here contains 4×10^6 cells (20 µg/DNA) in a total volume of 100 µL. Molds can be constructed in 0.5-mm perspex or tubing giving a total volume of 100 mm^3. It is advisable to leave the molds open-ended so that the plugs can be pushed out. Half the plug will contain approx 10 µg DNA and a quarter of the plug will contain 5 µg/mL DNA. Thus one plug can be used in more than one lane on the gel. When loading a section of the plug into the resolving gel care should be taken to ensure that it is in contact with both the bottom and the front of the well. Load all the plugs into the wells first and then seal with the molten agarose.

The isolation of large molecular weight DNA fragments from apoptotic cells using deproteinized agarose plugs, although straightforward, can be time-consuming and labor intensive. Walker et al. describe a method whereby sodium dodecylsulfate (SDS) lysates of apoptotic cells have been shown to be sufficiently deproteinized to run on either conventional or field inversion electrophoresis gels.

1×10^6 cells in 25-µL vol are added to an equal volume of 2% (w/v) SDS in Tris/EDTA/NaCl buffer. The resulting viscous lysate then is applied gently to wells, using pipet tips cut to a wide bore, and then kept in place with 1% low melting point agarose. Alternatively, the lysates can be mixed with equal volumes of agarose and formed into agarose plugs that are then applied and sealed into the resolving gel.

The electrophoresis unit for FIGE must be cooled actively. Overheating of the gel can be owing to a failure in the cooling system, e.g., the pump or the refrigeration unit, but an incorrect buffer formulation also can have the same effect.

References

1. Martin, S. J., Lennon, S. V., Bonham, A. M., and Cotter, T. G. (1990) Induction of apoptosis (programmed cell death) in human leukaemic HL-60 cells by inhibition of RNA or protein synthesis. *J. Immunol.* **145,** 1859–1867.
2. Filipski, J., Leblanc, J., Youdale, A., Sikorska, M., and Walker, P. R. (1990) Periodicity of DNA folding in higher order chromatin structures. *EMBO J.* **9,** 1319–1327.
3. Wood, A. C., Waters, C. M., Garner, A., and Hickman, J. A. (1994) Changes in c-myc expresssion and the kinetics of dexamethasone-induced programmed cell death (apoptosis) in human lymphoid leukaemia cells. *Br. J. Cancer* **69,** 663–669.
4. Walker, P. R., Smith, C., Youdale, A., Leblanc, J., Whitfield, J. F., and Sikorska, M. (1991) Topoisomerase II-reactive chemotherapeutic drugs induce apoptosis in thymocytes. *Cancer Res.* **51,** 1078–1085.
5. Walker, P. R., Kokileva, L., Leblanc, J., and Sikorska, M. (1993) Detection of the initial stages of DNA fragmentation in apoptosis. *BioTechniques* **15,** 1032–1040.
6. Schwartz, D. C. and Cantor, C. R. (1984) Separation of yeast chromosome-sized DNAs by pulsed field gradient gel electrophoresis. *Cell* **37,** 67–75.
7. Oberhammer, F., Wilson, J. W., Dive, C., Morris, I. D., Hickman, J. A., Wakeling, A. E., Walker, P. R., and Sikorska, M. (1993) Apoptotic death in epithelial cells:

cleavage of DNA to 300 and/or 50kb fragments prior to or in the absence of internucleosomal fragmentation. *EMBO J.* **12,** 3679–3684.

8. Brown, D. G., Sun, X.-M., and Cohen, G. M. (1993) Dexamethasone-induced apoptosis involves cleavage of DNA to large fragments prior to internucleosomal fragmentation. *J. Biol. Chem.* **268,** 3037–3039.

Further Reading

Kerr, J. F. R., Winterford, C. M., and Harmon, B. V. (1994) Apoptosis: its significance in cancer and cancer therapy. *Cancer* **73,** 2013–2026.

Smith, C. L. (ed.) (1993) Paper Symposium. Changing directions in electrophoresis. *Electrophoresis* **14,** 249–370.

Index

A

Alpha-satellite probe, 169
Aneusomy, 169
Antidigoxigenin-rhodamine, 163
Apoptosis, apoptotic ladders, 207
Autoradiographic detection, 151
Avidin-FITC, 163

B

β_2-microglobulin, 41
Bandshift, 134
Biotinylated anti-avidin, 163
Biotinylated primer, 12
Bone marrow transplantation (BMT), 105
   donor chimera, 105
   donor, 105
   graft versus leukemia, 105
   mixed chimera, 105
   protein polymorphisms, 106
   recipient, 105
Brophenol blue loading buffer, 52
BSA

C

cDNA synthesis, 30, 57
   PML-RAR-α cDNA synthesis, 50
Cell isolation
   mononuclear cell preparation, 28
     blood, 28
     bone marrow, 28
     bone marrow/blood cells, 43
       Ficoll, 43
Centromere probes, 167
Cesium chloride (CsC1) methods, 50
Chemiluminescence techniques, 116
Chloroform, 79
Chronic myeloid leukemia, 25
   Philadelphia (Ph) chromosome, 25
Citifluor glycerol mount, 163
Colcemid, 162

Comparative genomic hybridization (CGH), 183
   chromosome intensity profiles, 189
   clinically significant trisomies, 189
   color imbalance, 184
   deletion detection limit, 184
   DNA mixture preparation, 188
   genetic amplifications, 184
   genetic imbalance detection, 183
   image analysis, 188
   lymphomas, 183
   monosomies (13, 18, 21, X, Y), 189
   monsomy/trisomy detection, 183
   solid tumors, 183
   unbalanced translocations, 189
Constant field gel electrophoresis, 209
Contamination, 20
Cosmid, 169
Cot-1 DNA

D

DAPI, 163
   Antifade solution, 186
7-Deaza-dGTP, 137
Decon, 90, 163
Denaturing gradient gel electrophoresis (DGGE), 141
Densitometer, 97
(DEPC)-treated water, 79
Dextran sulfate, 162
DMSO, 80, 156
DNA, 3, 132
   clean up, Wizard PCR preps, 144
   elution of DNA, 10
     PAGE gels, 10
   extraction, storage
     archival material, 116
     blood smear, 117
     bone marrow, 68
     buccal wash, 109

extraction for CGH, 186
lymph node, 68
paraffin-embedded material, 116
slide, 68
stained slides, 117
labeling
CGH, 187
end labeling, 13
interpretation of results, 43
kinase labeling, 42
nonradioactive labeling, 44
PCR labeling, 155
radiolabeled, 152
quantification, 71
sequencer, 116
size marker, 52
φX1 ladder, 52
123-bp ladder, 52
100-bp ladder, 52
1-kb ladder, 52
DNase I, 172
dNTPs, 80
Dot blotting, 15
"drop-in" technique, 71
DTT, 80

E

Electroblot analysis, 15
false positive, 20
Escherichia coli DNA polymerase, 172
Ethidium bromide: Stock, 81

F

Field inversion gel electrophoresis (FIGE),
208
FIGE settings, 210
lauroyl sarcosine, 210
Fluorescent *in situ* hybridization (FISH),
92, 161
analysis for FISH, 176
bionick, 162
biotin, 171
biotin-11-dUTP, 171
biotin-16-dUTP, 171
biotin-14-dUTP, 171
biotin-11-dCTP, 171
bone marrow samples, 166
"citifluor," 175
confocal microscopy, 176

coplin jars, 174
counterstaining of slides, 175
DAPI banding, 188
denaturation and preparation of slides, 174
detection of posthybridization washes,
174
digital imaging, 176
digozigenin, 171
digoxigenin-11-dUTP, 171
dual-color hybridization, 177
EGR1, 100
FISH analysis, 99
herring sperm DNA, 162
hybridization, 171, 174
indirect method, 163
IRF1, 100
light microscopic analysis, 176
nick translation, 162
peripheral blood samples, 166
photometrics camera, 176
photometrics CCD camera, 176
posthybridization washes, 175
probe preparation, 162, 167
rehybridization, 171
signal detection, 175
slide preparation, 166
smartCapture software, 176
Formamide, 162

G

γ^{32}P dATP, 81
Gel electrophoresis
agarose, 133
"mini" gel, 209
Gel/running conditions, 156
Genes
AF-4 gene, 61
AF-9, 61
AF-X, 61
ALL-1, 55
all-trans retinoic acid, 47
APC gene, 100
BCL-2, 63, 207
BCL6/LAZ3, 76
BCR-ABL
AML-M2, 37
AML1, 37
AML1/ETO, 43
ETO gene, 37

MTG8, 37
  p210, 26
  p190, 26
  transcripts, 26
bcr types 1 or 2, 50
c-myc, 207
ENL, 61
HRX, 55
HTRX, 55
MCC gene, 100
MLL gene, 55
non-Hodgkin's lymphoma (NHL), 75
NPM-ALK fusion gene, 76
NPM-AL, 78
p53, 207
PML/RAR, 47
retinoblastoma (RBI)
  mutations, 123
  mutations incidence, 138
Wilms' tumor (WT1), 141
WT1 mutations, 146
Gene dosage analysis, 97
Gene loss, Quantitative assessment, 97
Glass wool, 187
Glycerol in the gel, 156

H

Hanks balanced salt solution (HBSS), 209
Heterozygosity, 97

I

Immunoglobulin heavy chain (IgH), 3
  IgH probes, 12
  probe design, 13
    DNJ sequence, 14
    junctional sequence, 13
In situ hybridization (ISH), 193
  autoradiography, 203
  development of slides, 203
  hybridization and washing sections, 201
  photography, 205
  prehybridization, 201
  preparation of probes, 196
  slide and coverslip preparation, 199
  ^{35}S-radiolabeled probe, 197
  synthesis of single-stranded RNA
    probes, 198
  tissue fixation, embedding and
    sectioning, 199

Isoamyl alcohol, 79
Isopropanol, 79
Interphase cells, 161, 169

K

Ki-1 (CD30), 76

L

Leukemia, APL, 49
Linkage analysis, 123
Locus-specific probes, 169

M

Magnetic particle separator, 12
Metaphase analysis, 161
Methanol: glacial acid fixative, 162
Microsatellite polymorphisms, 96
Mineral oil, 156
Minimal residual disease (MRD), 3, 44
Myelodysplastic syndrome
  5q-syndrome
  Genes
    CSF1R gene, 91
    CSF2, 92
    EGR1, 92
    FGFA gene, 91
    IL9, 92
    IL5, 92
    NKSF1 gene, 91
    tumor suppressor gene, 91

N

Nick translation, 172
Nondenaturing gels
  preparation, 133
PCR, 10
  clone-specific, 10
  cycler parameters, 10
  DOP-PCR, 167
  IgH, 10
  PCR reaction mixture store, 52
  PCR remission samples, 14
    allele-specific hybridization, 15
PML/RAR
  controls, 52
  sensitivity, 66
t(14;18)
  oligonucleotides, 68
  primers, 68

Phage, 169
Phenol, 79
Phytohemagglutinin (PHA), 162
Premature stop codons, 138
Proteinase K/CaCl2, 163
Propidium iodide, 163
Purification of single-stranded DNA, 135

R

Random hexamers, 48
Restriction enzyme digestion PCR products, 133
Restriction fragment length polymorphism (RFLP), 92, 106
  PCR
    dinucleotide repeats, 96
    tetronucleotide repeats, 96
    trinucleotide repeats, 96
Reverse transcriptase, 80
Ribonuclease A, 209
RNA
  isolation of mRNA, 59
  RNA extraction, 28, 49, 81
  RNA isolation, 57
RNase protection, 151
RNasin, 80
RT-PCR, 25
  AML1/ETO, 41
  β_2-microglobulin, 42
  BCR-ABL, 25
    multiplex PCR, 30
    nested PCR, 26, 30, 50
    quantitative PCR, 31
    PCR contamination, 31
  PML-RAR-α, 50
  t (2;5), 80

S

Safety precautions, 152
SDS, 81
Sephadex G-50 column, 71, 186
Sequenase, 144

Sequencing,
  acrylamide gel porosity, 157
  cycle sequencing, 13
  fixation of the gel, 157
  gel dimensions, 157
Single-strand conformation polymorphism analysis (SSCP), 123
SSC, 81
STE, 135
Streptavidin-coated beads, 135
Southern analysis, 95
Southern blotting, 42

T

T-cell receptor (TCR), 3
  ALL, 3
T4 polynucleotide kinase, 81
Taq DNA polymerase, 80
Texas Red-dUTP, 186
Translocation t(14;18), 63
  benign hyperplastic tonsils, 65
  blood donors, 65
  Hodgkin's disease, 65
  immunoblastic lymphoma, 65
  large cell lymphoma, 65
  MBR, 63
  MCR, 64
  "N" regions, 64
Tris borate electrophoresis buffer (TBE), 81
Tween-20, 162

U

Ultra violet irradiation, 82

V

Variable number tandem repeats (VNTRs), 106

W

Whole chromosome paints, 167

Y

Yeast artificial chromosomes, 167, 169